Haematology

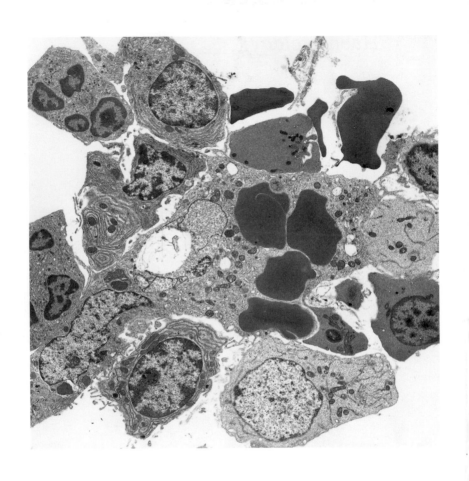

Contents

Colour plates 1–48 appear between pages 152 and 153

Preface to the Sixth Edition

In the 5 years since the publication of the fifth edition, there have been considerable advances in our understanding of the molecular biology and pathogenesis of a number of haematological disorders together with further advances in therapy. The present edition has been extensively revised and updated to incorporate these developments, whilst constantly keeping sight of the fact that it is primarily written to provide core haematological knowledge required by a medical student. A new feature of this edition is that non-core information, supplied to enhance understanding, is boxed and printed in smaller type so that it is clearly distinguished from the core text. As in previous editions, the book aims to integrate the physiological, pathological and clinical aspects of haematology and, wherever possible, to avoid the presentation of tedious lists of unexplained facts. The emphasis is to provide a sound understanding of essential principles. Chapters 1–12 begin with a list of objectives in learning in order to help undergraduates when learning the subject and when revising for examinations.

We thank Miss Gale Lewis for her tireless secretarial help and for assistance with proof reading.

N. C. Hughes-Jones
S. N. Wickramasinghe

Acknowledgements

We are grateful to Bio Products Laboratory of the UK NHS National Blood Authority and Roche Products Limited for generously sponsoring the colour plates.

Preface to the First Edition

These lecture notes are designed to supply the basic knowledge of both the clinical and laboratory aspects of haematological diseases and blood transfusion. The content is broadly similar to that of the course given to medical students by the Department of Haematology at St Mary's Hospital Medical School. References have been cited so that those who need to extend their knowledge in any particular field can do so. Most of the journals and books that are mentioned are those commonly found in every library.

At the end of each chapter I have supplied a list of objectives in studying each disease. There are two main purposes in these objectives. First, they facilitate the learning process, since the process of acquisition, retention and recall of data is greatly helped if the facts and concepts are centred around a particular objective. Secondly, many objectives are closely related to the practical problems encountered in the diagnosis and treatment of patients. For instance, the following objectives: 'to understand the method of differentiation of megaloblastic anaemia due to vitamin B_{12} deficiency from that due to folate deficiency' and 'to understand the basis for the differentiation of leukaemia into acute and chronic forms based on the clinical picture and on the peripheral blood findings' are practical problems encountered frequently in the haematology laboratory. A point of more immediate interest to the undergraduate is that examiners setting either multiple choice or essay questions will be searching for the same knowledge that is required in answering the objectives.

I should like to thank Professor P. L. Mollison, Dr P. Barkhan, Dr I. Chanarin, Dr G. J. Jenkins and Dr M. S. Rose for their criticism and helpful suggestions during the preparation of the manuscript and Mrs Inge Barnett for typing the several drafts and final typescript.

N. C. Hughes-Jones

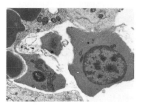

Normal Haemoglobin, Blood Cells and Haemopoiesis

Objectives in learning

1 To have a basic understanding of the structure and functions of the haemoglobin molecule.

2 To know about the general features of globin genes – their location, structure, transcription and translation.

3 To be able to identify the various types of normal blood cells in colour transparencies or photographs.

4 To know the functions, concentration and life-span of various types of blood cell.

5 To understand the concept of a stem cell.

6 To understand how blood cells are produced from pluripotent haemopoietic stem cells and how haemopoiesis is regulated.

7 To be able to identify erythroblasts, neutrophil precursors and megakaryocytes in colour transparencies or photographs.

8 To be aware of differences in the sites of haemopoiesis during human development and the reappearance of extramedullary haemopoiesis in some haematological disorders.

Normal haemoglobin and its synthesis

STRUCTURE AND FUNCTION

Normal human haemoglobins (Hbs) are tetramers consisting of two pairs of unlike globin chains; each of the four chains is associated with one haem group located within a hydrophobic crevice. In adult Hbs, α-chains are associated mainly with β-chains (HbA; $\alpha_2\beta_2$) and to a much lesser extent with δ-chains (HbA$_2$; $\alpha_2\delta_2$). In fetal Hb, α-chains are associated with γ-chains (HbF; $\alpha_2\gamma_2$). In the embryonic Hbs, ζ-chains are associated with ε-chains (Hb Gower 1; $\zeta_2\varepsilon_2$) or γ-chains (Hb Portland; $\zeta_2\gamma_2$) and α-chains are associated with ε-chains (Hb Gower 2; $\alpha_2\varepsilon_2$). There are two types of γ-chains in HbF which differ only in the amino acid at position 136, which may be glycine ($^G\gamma$ chains) or alanine ($^A\gamma$ chains).

When the percentage O_2 saturation of Hb at various O_2 tensions (in mmHg) is determined in the laboratory and the two values are plotted against each other, a sigmoid O_2 dissociation (O_2 affinity) curve is obtained (Fig. 1.1). This is because the binding of one O_2 molecule to the haem group on one globin chain of the tetrameric Hb molecule promotes the binding of the next O_2 molecule to the haem group on another globin chain. This haem—haem interaction results from a small shape change in the molecule that occurs when O_2 combines with haem. In the deoxygenated state, the two β-chains are separated slightly such that one molecule of 2,3-diphosphoglycerate (2,3-DPG) can enter the Hb molecule and bind to the β-chains; in the oxygenated state, the 2,3-DPG is ejected. The partial pressure of O_2 at which normal Hb is half-saturated with O_2 (P_{50}) is 26 mmHg (at pH 7.4, 37°C). *In vivo*, exchange of O_2 normally occurs between a Po_2 of 95 mmHg (95% saturation) in arterial blood and a Po_2 of 40 mmHg (70% saturation) in venous blood.

The O_2 affinity of Hb is decreased (O_2 dissociation curve shifted to the right) by an increase in the amount of CO_2 in blood (Bohr effect). The CO_2 generates hydrogen ions by reacting with water, and the reduced O_2 affinity results from the combination of hydrogen ions with deoxyhaemoglobin; these hydrogen ions are released when Hb is oxygenated. Thus the Bohr effect facilitates release of O_2 in tissues and the unloading of CO_2 in the lungs. A second mechanism by which CO_2 generated in tissues decreases the O_2 affinity of Hb (i.e. facilitates release of O_2) is by reacting with the amino groups of the α-globin chains to form

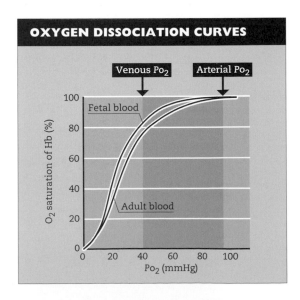

Fig. 1.1 Oxygen dissociation curves of human blood.

carbamates. When Hb combines with O_2 in the alveoli, this CO_2 is released.

The O_2 affinity of Hb is increased by a decrease in 2,3-DPG levels as occurs in stored blood, and decreased by an increase in 2,3-DPG levels as occurs in hypoxia. The O_2 affinity of HbF is higher than that of HbA because γ-chains bind to 2,3-DPG more weakly than β-chains. The high affinity of HbF facilitates O_2 transport from mother to fetus. O_2 affinity is decreased by an increase in body temperature (e.g. during fever).

SYNTHESIS

The genes for the ε-, $^G\gamma$-, $^A\gamma$-, δ- and β-chains are found in this order (5' to 3') in a linked cluster on chromosome 11. The α gene is duplicated so that there are two α genes close to the ζ gene on chromosome 16 in the linkage order ζ, $\alpha 2$, $\alpha 1$ (5' to 3'). Interestingly, in both chromosomes 11 and 16, the genes are arranged in the order in which they are switched on during intrauterine life.

There are a number of conserved sequences in the upstream flanking regions of the globin genes. Such sequences are involved in the regulation of globin gene expression and are known as promoters. They include: (a) the TATA box; and (b) two elements further upstream, the CCAAT box and CACCC and/or CCGCCC motifs. These promoters are recognized by non-specific, tissue-specific, and possibly developmental stage-restricted transcription factors that are involved in the attachment and correct positioning of the transcription initiation complex, which includes RNA polymerase (the enzyme involved in mRNA synthesis), at the TATA box. The globin gene promoters (except the α-gene promoter) include a recognition site (A/TGATAA/G) for the transacting erythroid-specific regulator known as GATA-1. Expression of genes in the entire β-globin gene cluster is influenced by a remote regulatory region known as the β-locus control region (β-LCR), which is situated upstream of the ε gene. Expression of genes in the entire α-globin gene cluster is controlled by a regulatory element known as HS-40 located upstream of the ζ gene.

Each globin gene contains two non-coding regions, also known as intervening sequences (IVS) or introns (i.e. regions that are not represented in the mature mRNA) and three coding regions or exons (Fig. 1.2). The initial mRNA transcript (mRNA precursor) is large and complementary to all regions (coding and non-coding) of the globin gene, but the regions complementary to the base sequences of the introns are soon removed by excision and ligation (spliced) and are absent in the mature mRNA. Within the nucleus, the mRNA is modified at the 5' end by the formation of a CAP structure and stabilized by polyadenylation at the 3'

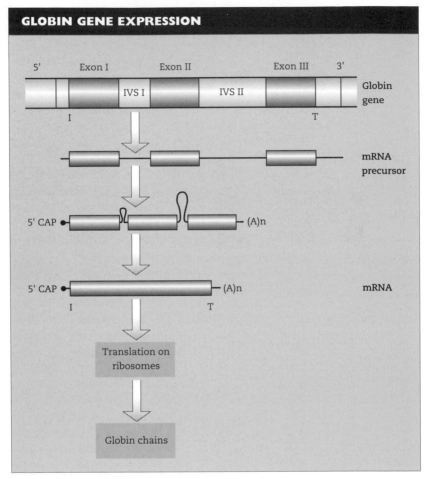

Fig. 1.2 Expression of globin genes. IVS, intervening sequence; I, initiator codon; T, termination codon; (A)n, polyadenylation site; 5′ CAP, structure containing 7-methyl guanosine.

end. The mature mRNA enters the cytoplasm and attaches to ribosomes on which globin chain synthesis (translation) occurs.

Blood cells

MORPHOLOGY

On Romanowsky-stained blood smears, normal erythrocytes appear as red, anucleate cells with circular outlines and have diameters between

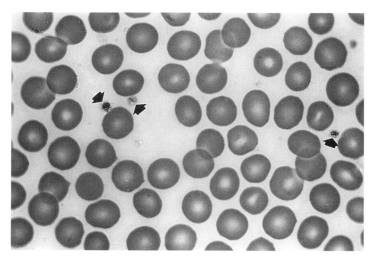

Fig. 1.3 Smear of normal peripheral venous blood. The red cells are round and do not vary greatly in size. They are well-filled with haemoglobin; the central area of pallor is small. A few platelets (arrowed) are also present.

6.7 and 7.7 μm (mean 7.2 μm). Blood-cell morphology should be assessed in a region of the blood smear in which only occasional red cells overlap. In such a region, each red cell (which is biconcave in shape) has a central area of pallor whose diameter is about a third of the red-cell diameter (Fig. 1.3).

In addition to red cells, blood smears contain platelets and various types of white cell. On average, the ratio between red cells, platelets and leucocytes is 700:40:1. The platelets are small anucleate cells, about 2–3 μm in diameter (Fig. 1.3). They stain light blue and contain a number of small azurophilic granules which are often concentrated at the centre. The important features of the morphology of normal leucocytes are summarized in Table 1.1. Neutrophil, eosinophil and basophil granulocytes (Fig. 1.4; Plates 1, 2 and 4) are also described as polymorphonuclear leucocytes or polymorphs: the two or more nuclear masses in each cell are joined in series by fine strands of nuclear chromatin. Normally, the proportion of neutrophil polymorphs with five or more nuclear segments is 3% or less. Monocytes from the peripheral blood of a normal adult are shown in Fig. 1.5 and Plate 4. Small lymphocytes (Fig. 1.5; Plate 3) account for about 90% of lymphocytes in the blood; large lymphocytes for the remaining 10%.

NUMBER AND LIFE-SPAN
The reference ranges for concentrations of various types of blood cell in

WHITE CELL MORPHOLOGY

| Cell type | Cell size (μm) | Cytoplasm | | | Nucleus |
		Colour	Ratio of cytoplasmic volume to nuclear volume	Granules	
Neutrophil granulocytes	9–15	Slightly pink	High	Numerous, very fine, faint purple	Usually two to five segments
Eosinophil granulocytes	12–17	Pale blue	High	Many, large and rounded, reddish-orange	Usually two segments
Basophil granulocytes	10–14		High	Several, large and rounded, dark purplish-black	Usually two segments, granules overlie nucleus
Monocytes	15–30	Pale greyish-blue, cytoplasmic vacuoles may be seen	Moderately high or high	Variable number, fine, purplish-red	Various shapes (rounded, C- or U-shaped, lobulated), skein-like or lacy chromatin
Lymphocytes	7–12 (small lymphocytes); 12–16 (large lymphocytes)	Pale blue	Low or very low	Few, fine purplish-red	Rounded with large clumps of condensed chromatin

Table 1.1 Morphology of normal white cells in Romanowsky-stained smears of peripheral blood.

(a) 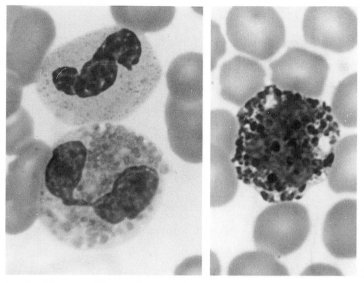 (b)

Fig. 1.4 (a) Neutrophil granulocyte and eosinophil granulocyte. (b) Basophil granulocyte.

adults are given in Table 1.2, together with data on their life-span in the blood. Ranges for the Hb and packed cell volume (PCV) in healthy individuals are given on p. 25. Normal red cells circulate for 110–120 days and at the end of their life-span are phagocytosed in the bone marrow, spleen and liver by macrophages (a component of the reticuloendothelial system). The neutrophil granulocytes in the blood are distributed between a marginated granulocyte pool (consisting of cells that are loosely attached to the endothelial lining of small venules) and a circulating granulocyte pool. There is a continuous exchange of cells between these two pools and in healthy subjects, the circulating granulocyte pool accounts for between 16 and 99% (average, 44%) of all blood granulocytes. When cell counts are determined on samples of peripheral venous blood, only the circulating granulocytes are being studied. In healthy Caucasian adults, the reference range for the absolute neutrophil count is $1.5–7.5 \times 10^9/l$. The lower limit for the reference range is lower in healthy Blacks, being about $1.0 \times 10^9/l$. Neutrophil granulocytes leave the circulation exponentially, with an average $t_{1/2}$ of about 7 hours, and probably survive in tissues and secretions for about another 30 hours.

Lymphocytes continuously recirculate between the blood and lymphatic system. They leave the blood between the endothelial cells of the

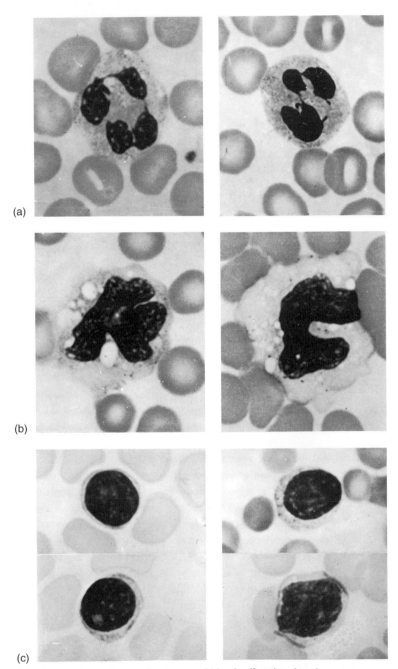

Fig. 1.5 Photomicrographs of normal blood cells printed at the same magnification. (a) Two neutrophil granulocytes. (b) Two monocytes. (c) Four lymphocytes of various sizes.

CONCENTRATION AND LIFE-SPAN OF BLOOD CELLS

Cell type	Reference range (95% reference limits)	Life-span in blood
Red cells	Males 4.4–5.8 × 10^{12}/l Females 4.1–5.2 × 10^{12}/l	110–120 days
White cells (leucocytes)	4.0–11.0 × 10^9/l*	
Neutrophil granulocytes	1.5–7.5 × 10^9/l*	$t_{1/2}$ approx. 7 hours
Eosinophil granulocytes	0.02–0.60 × 10^9/l	$t_{1/2}$ approx. 6 hours
Basophil granulocytes	0.01–0.15 × 10^9/l	
Monocytes	0.2–0.8 × 10^9/l	$t_{1/2}$ approx. 70 hours
Lymphocytes	1.2–3.5 × 10^9/l	
Platelets	160–450 × 10^9/l	9–12 days

* Applies to Caucasians.

Table 1.2 Ninety five per cent reference limits for the concentrations of various types of circulating blood cell in adults and their life-span in the blood.

post-capillary venules of lymph nodes, migrate through the lymph node into efferent lymphatics and re-enter the blood via the thoracic duct. The majority of human lymphocytes are long-lived, with average life-spans of 4–5 years and maximum life-spans greater than 20 years. The short-lived lymphocytes survive for about 3 days.

FUNCTIONS

The main functions of blood cells are summarized in Table 1.3. More details of platelet function are given on pp. 205 and 206.

Neutrophils and monocytes

Monocytes are the precursors of tissue macrophages. Phagocytosis of microorganisms and cells coated with antibody (with their exposed Fc fragments) and complement (especially C3b) occurs via binding to Fc and C3b receptors on the surface of neutrophils, monocytes

BLOOD CELL FUNCTIONS

Type of cell	Main functions
Red blood cells (erythrocytes)	Transport O_2 from lungs to tissues; transport CO_2 from tissues to lungs (see p. 2)
Neutrophil granulocytes	Chemotaxis, phagocytosis, killing of phagocytosed bacteria
Eosinophil granulocytes	All neutrophil functions listed above, effector cells for antibody-dependent damage to metazoal parasites, regulate immediate-type hypersensitivity reactions (inactivate histamine and leukotrienes released by basophils and mast cells)
Basophil granulocytes	Mediate immediate-type hypersensitivity (IgE-coated basophils react with specific antigen and release histamine and leukotrienes), modulate inflammatory responses by releasing heparin and proteases
Monocytes (and macrophages*)	Chemotaxis, phagocytosis, killing of some microorganisms, antigen presentation, release of IL-1 and TNF which stimulate bone marrow stromal cells to produce GM-CSF, G-CSF, M-CSF and IL-6 (p. 20)
Platelets	Adhere to subendothelial connective tissue, participate in blood clotting (see p. 205)
Lymphocytes	Involved in immune responses and production of haemopoietic growth factors (p. 12)

* Macrophages are tissue cells derived from monocytes.

Table 1.3 Main functions of blood cells.

and macrophages. Bacteria and fungi that are not antibody-coated are phagocytosed after binding to mannose receptors on the phagocyte surface. The killing of phagocytosed microorganisms involves O_2-dependent and O_2-independent mechanisms.

The superoxide-dependent microbicidal agents include H_2O_2, hypochlorous acid, chloramines and hydroxyl radicals (OH·). Superoxide (O_2^-) is produced by neutrophils and some γ-interferon-stimulated macrophages during the respiratory burst which follows their activation and lasts from a few seconds to 15 minutes. The generation of O_2^-
Continued

results from the reduction of O_2 by NADPH, which is catalysed by membrane-bound respiratory burst oxidase, one component of which is cytochrome b_{558}. The O_2^- undergoes dismutation to O_2 and H_2O_2. It also generates hydroxyl radicals by reaction with H_2O_2. Myeloperoxidase, found in the primary granules of neutrophils, catalyses the formation of the strong microbicidal agent hypochlorous acid from Cl^- and H_2O_2. The hypochlorous acid so formed reacts with amines to form chloramines.

Non-O_2-dependent microbicidal mechanisms include a reduction of pH within phagocytic vacuoles (phagosomes) and the release into phagosomes of: (a) lysozyme (found within azurophilic and specific granules), which causes swelling and rupture of bacteria; and (b) the iron-binding protein lactoferrin, which may prevent ingested bacteria from taking up iron.

Note Throughout text, boxed type is non-core: provided only to enhance understanding.

Lymphocytes

Between 65 and 80% of peripheral blood lymphocytes are T cells, 10–30% are B cells and 2–10% are non-T and non-B cells (null cells). Both B and T cells are formed with specific antigen-recognizing molecules on their cell surface which determine that each cell recognizes a specific antigenic determinant. The antigen-recognizing molecules for B and T cells are, respectively, immunoglobulin and the T-cell receptor molecule. The cells are triggered into proliferation when they react with the specific antigen in the presence of appropriate accessory cells; their progeny develop into effector cells or memory cells.

The effector T-lymphocytes include helper cells (CD4-positive cells), which promote the function of B cells and are required for the maturation of other types of T cell, and suppressor-cytotoxic cells (CD8-positive cells) which inhibit the function of other lymphocytes and are cytotoxic towards foreign and virus-infected cells. The ratio of helper to suppressor cells is 1.5–2.5 : 1. The null cells include killer (K) cells and natural killer (NK) cells. The killer cells lyse antibody-coated target cells and are therefore also called antibody-dependent cytotoxic cells (ADCC). The NK cells kill tumour cells and virus-infected cells in the absence of antibody. Thus, the functions of the T cells include:

1   mediation of cellular immunity against viruses, fungi and low-grade intracellular pathogens such as mycobacteria;

2   participation in delayed hypersensitivity reactions, tumour rejection and graft rejection;

3 interaction with B cells in producing antibodies against certain antigens, and

4 suppression of B-cell function.

Activated T cells also produce IL-5 (eosinophil colony-stimulating factor) which is involved in the regulation of eosinophil granulocytopoiesis and IL-3, one of the multilineage haemopoietic growth factors. (This explains the excessive eosinophil production in some T-cell lymphomas.) They also produce other haemopoietic growth factors (interleukin-6 (IL-6), granulocyte-macrophage colony-stimulating factor (GM-CSF), granulocyte colony-stimulating factor (G-CSF), macrophage colony-stimulating factor (M-CSF)) (p. 20).

The percentages of B cells that express IgM, IgD, IgG and IgA molecules on their surface are, respectively, 40, 30, 30 and 10. Many B cells have both IgM and IgD on their surface but others usually have only IgG or IgA. A single B cell expresses immunoglobulins of only one light chain type, and there are twice as many cells with $\varkappa$ light chains as there are with λ light chains. B cells that are activated by reaction with a specific antigen develop into antibody-secreting plasma cells or into B-memory cells. Most of the antibodies formed during a primary antibody response consist of IgM, and almost all of the antibodies formed during a secondary antibody response (which results from the activation of B-memory cells) consist of IgG.

Haemopoiesis in the adult

In normal adults, haemopoiesis (production of blood cells) only occurs in the marrow contained within certain bones (p. 22).

GENERAL CONSIDERATIONS AND EARLY EVENTS

Haemopoietic systems of adults are examples of steady-state cell renewal systems in which the rate of loss of mature cells (red cells, granulocytes, monocytes, lymphocytes and platelets) from the blood is balanced fairly precisely by the rate of release of newly formed cells into the blood. Mature cells are lost either because of ageing or during the performance of normal functions.

The formation of blood cells involves two processes:

1 progressive development of structural and functional characteristics specific for a given cell type (cytodifferentiation or maturation), and

2 cell proliferation.

A schematic representation of haemopoiesis is shown in Fig. 1.6. The stem cells and progenitor cells are involved early in haemopoiesis; they cannot be recognized morphologically in marrow smears but can be

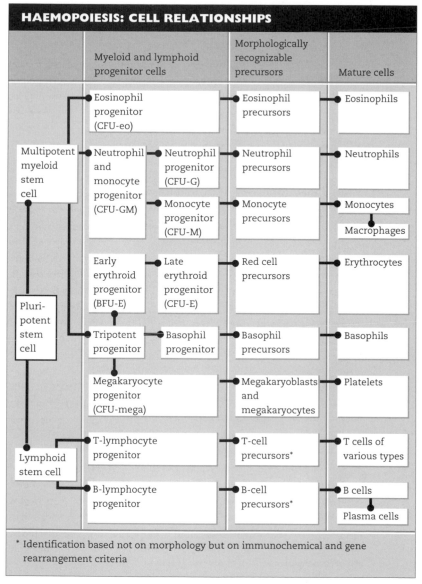

Fig. 1.6 Relationships between the various types of cell involved in haemopoiesis.

studied by functional tests. In man, these cells (colony-forming units or CFU) have been identified and characterized on the basis of their ability to produce small colonies of one or more cell types when grown in semi-solid media containing appropriate haemopoietic growth factors. The most primitive haemopoietic cell is the pluripotent haemopoietic stem cell. This gives rise to two types of committed stem cell, namely multipotent myeloid stem cells and lymphoid stem cells. The essential characteristics of stem cells are:

I   an extensive capacity to maintain their own number by cell proliferation, and

2   the capacity to mature into other cell types.

The lymphoid stem cells give rise to lymphocyte progenitor cells that eventually mature into all types of T, B and non-T, non-B lymphocytes. The multipotent myeloid stem cells differentiate into various types of myeloid progenitor cell which eventually generate erythrocytes, neutrophils, eosinophils, basophils and mast cells, monocytes and plate-lets. *Unlike the stem cells, the lymphoid and myeloid progenitor cells have only a limited capacity for self-renewal.*

The more immature myeloid progenitor cells are committed to two or three differentiation pathways. With increasing maturity, their differentiation potential becomes progressively limited, eventually to one pathway only. The unipotent progenitor cells committed to the production of erythrocytes, neutrophil granulocytes, monocytes/macrophages and megakaryocytes are, respectively, called CFU-E, CFU-G, CFU-M and CFU-mega. They mature into the earliest morphologically recognizable cells of the corresponding cell lineage (pronormoblasts, myeloblasts, monoblasts and megakaryoblasts).

Stem cells account for about I per 10 000–100 000 nucleated marrow cells. They are also found in very small numbers in circulating blood so that stem cells used for marrow transplantation can be derived not only from bone marrow but also from peripheral blood. Haemopoietic progenitor cells are also found both in marrow and in blood. Despite their presence in blood, myeloid stem cells and progenitor cells normally develop into morphologically recognizable haemopoietic cells only within the microenvironment of the bone marrow.

MORPHOLOGICALLY RECOGNIZABLE HAEMOPOIETIC CELLS DERIVED FROM MYELOID STEM CELLS

In every myeloid cell lineage other than that involved in platelet production, the early precursors that can be identified on morphological and cytochemical criteria are capable of both dividing and maturing. The late precursors do not divide but continue to mature. The proliferative activity during haemopoiesis serves as an amplifying mechanism and ensures that a large number of mature blood cells are derived from a single cell that becomes committed to any particular lineage.

Erythropoiesis

The pronormoblast is a large cell with a small quantity of agranular intensely basophilic cytoplasm (due to the presence of numerous ribosomes) and a large nucleus containing finely dispersed nuclear chromatin and nucleoli (Fig. 1.7a). The successive stages through which a pronormoblast develops into erythrocytes are termed basophilic normoblasts (Fig. 1.7b); early and late polychromatic normoblasts (Fig. 1.7c,d); marrow reticulocytes and blood reticulocytes. Nucleated cell

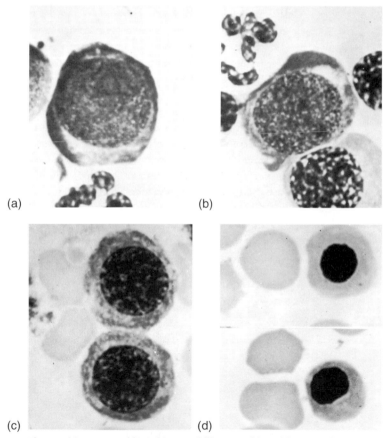

(a)   (b)   (c)   (d)

Fig. 1.7 (a) Pronormoblast. (b) Basophilic normoblast. (c) Two early polychromatic normoblasts. (d) Two late polychromatic normoblasts. The granules of condensed chromatin in the basophilic normoblast are slightly coarser than in the pronormoblast. The nuclei of the late polychromatic normoblasts contain large masses of condensed chromatin.

classes of increasing maturity show: (a) a progressive reduction in cell and nuclear size; (b) a progressive increase in the quantity of condensed nuclear chromatin; (c) a progressive increase in the ratio of cytoplasmic volume to nuclear volume; and (d) a progressive increase in Hb (which stains pink) and a progressive decrease in ribosomal RNA (which stains blue), resulting in polychromasia (grey-pink colour). The late polychromatic normoblast extrudes its nucleus and becomes a marrow reticulocyte. The marrow reticulocytes enter the blood stream and circulate for 1–2 days before becoming mature red cells.

In Romanowsky-stained marrow and blood smears, reticulocytes appear as rounded, faintly polychromatic cells whose diameters are slightly larger than those of mature red cells. When living polychromatic red cells are incubated with brilliant cresyl blue (supravital staining), the ribosomes form a basophilic precipitate of granules or filaments or both; in the most immature of these cells the precipitated RNA appears as a basophilic reticulum (hence the term reticulocyte) (Fig. 1.8). Mature red cells lack ribosomes.

On the basis of their morphological features, nucleated red-cell precursors (erythroblasts) found in normal marrow are called normoblasts and normal erythropoiesis is described as being normoblastic in type. The characteristic feature of normoblastic erythropoiesis is the presence of moderate quantities of condensed nuclear chromatin in early polychromatic erythroblasts. Even in healthy individuals, a few erythroblasts fail to develop normally and such cells are recognized and phagocytosed by bone marrow macrophages. This loss of potential

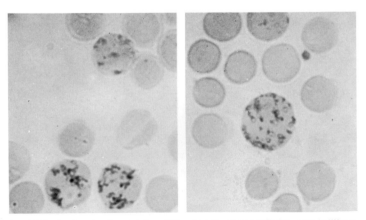

Fig. 1.8 Reticulocytes in peripheral blood stained supravitally with brilliant cresyl blue. Note the reticulum of precipitated ribosomes.

erythrocytes due to the intramedullary destruction of red-cell precursors is described as ineffective erythropoiesis. The extent of ineffective erythropoiesis in normal marrow is slight.

Neutrophil granulocytopoiesis

The myeloblasts superficially resemble pronormoblasts except that their cytoplasm is less basophilic. The successive cytological classes through which a myeloblast matures into circulating neutrophil granulocytes are termed promyelocytes, neutrophil myelocytes, neutrophil metamyelocytes, neutrophil band cells (stab cells) and neutrophil granulocytes (Fig. 1.9, Plates 7–9). During this maturation the following changes occur:

1   a progressive reduction of cytoplasmic basophilia and a progressive increase in the quantity of condensed chromatin after the promyelocyte stage;

2   the formation of coarse purplish-red (azurophilic) cytoplasmic granules (primary granules) at the promyelocyte stage, which remain visible at the myelocyte stage but not later;

3   the formation of fine neutrophilic granules (specific granules) at the myelocyte and metamyelocyte stages;

4   indentation of the nucleus which is moderate at the metamyelocyte stage (C-shaped nucleus) and more marked at the band cell stage (U-shaped, curved or coiled band-like nucleus), and

5   progressive segmentation of the U-shaped or band-like nucleus of the band cell leading to the formation of granulocytes with two to five nuclear lobes.

Megakaryocytopoiesis

During megakaryocytopoiesis, there is replication of DNA without nuclear or cell division which leads to the generation of very large uninucleate cells with DNA contents between 8c and 64c (other haemopoietic cells have DNA contents between 2c and 4c; 1c is the DNA content of a germ cell). There is a rough correlation between the DNA content of a megakaryocyte nucleus and both its size and extent of lobulation. A mature megakaryocyte is illustrated in Fig. 1.10 and in Plate 10. Large numbers of platelets are formed from the cytoplasm of each mature megakaryocyte; these are rapidly discharged directly into the marrow sinusoids. The residual 'bare' megakaryocyte nucleus is phagocytosed by macrophages.

Monocytopoiesis

The cell classes belonging to the monocyte–macrophage lineage

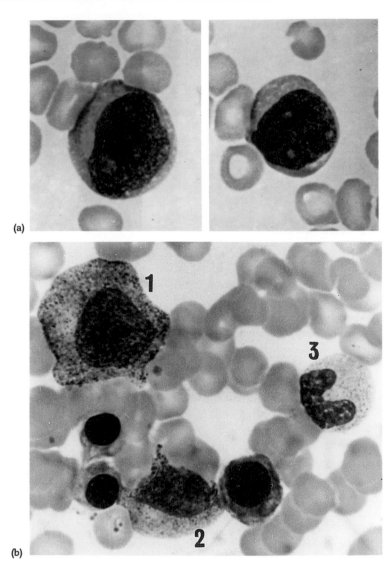

(a)

(b)

Fig. 1.9 Neutrophil precursors from normal bone marrow. (a) Two myeloblasts. (b) Promyelocyte (1), myelocyte (2) and metamyelocyte (3).

(mononuclear phagocyte system) are, in increasing order of maturity: monoblasts, promonocytes, marrow monocytes, blood monocytes and tissue macrophages.

LYMPHOCYTOPOIESIS

The lymphoid stem cell in the bone marrow generates B-cell progenitors

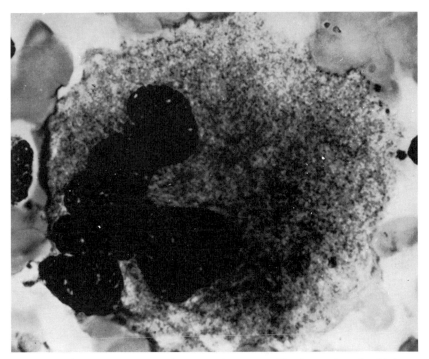

Fig. 1.10 Mature megakaryocyte (same magnification as Fig. 1.9). This is a very large cell with a single lobulated nucleus. Compare the size of the megakaryocyte with that of the erythroblasts in Fig. 1.9.

within that tissue. The B-cell progenitors undergo maturation into B cells in the microenvironment of the marrow and then travel via the blood into the B-cell zones of peripheral lymphoid tissue (follicles and medulla of lymph nodes and splenic follicles).

Either the lymphoid stem cells or primitive T-cell progenitors derived from them migrate from the marrow, via the blood, into the thymus where maturation into T cells takes place; those T cells which recognize self are deleted. The T cells later migrate to the T-cell zones of peripheral lymphoid organs (paracortical areas and medulla of lymph nodes and periarteriolar lymphoid sheaths of the spleen).

The terms used to describe cells at various stages of B-lymphocyte differentiation in the bone marrow and T-lymphocyte differentiation in the thymus are as follows:

Early pre-B cell → pre-B cell → immature B cell → mature B cell

Pre-T cell (thymic lymphoblast) → early thymocyte (large cortical thymocyte) → intermediate thymocyte (small cortical thymocyte) → late thymocyte (medullary thymocyte) → mature T cell.

All these stages have the morphological features of either lymphoblasts or lymphocytes. The identification of different lymphocyte precursors is therefore based not on morphology but on various properties like reactivity with certain monoclonal antibodies, immunoglobulin gene rearrangement status, presence of immunoglobulin on the surface membrane, presence of μ-chains or immunoglobulin within the cytoplasm, terminal deoxynucleotidyl-transferase (TdT) activity and T-cell receptor gene rearrangement status (Tables 1.4 and 1.5).

REGULATION OF HAEMOPOIESIS

The regulation of haemopoietic stem cells seems to depend on:

1   intimate contact with one or more types of bone marrow stromal cell (macrophages, T-lymphocytes, endothelial cells and fibroblasts) and components of the extracellular matrix, and

2   the haemopoietic growth factor known as the stem cell factor (SCF, kit ligand or Steel factor) produced by stromal cells.

The proliferation and maturation of both the early and the lineage committed bi- or unipotent progenitor cells are influenced by a number of haemopoietic growth factors secreted by stromal cells. These include the multilineage growth factors SCF, interleukin-3 (IL-3) and GM-CSF, and the more lineage-specific growth factors such as G-CSF, M-CSF, IL-5 (influencing CFUeo), thrombopoietin (influencing CFUmega) and erythropoietin. These growth factors react with specific receptors on the cell membrane of target cells and mediate their effects on survival, proliferation and differentiation via second messengers. In their absence, the target cell undergoes programmed cell death (apoptosis). All the haemopoietic growth factors are glycoproteins and some (erythropoietin, GM-CSF, G-CSF) have been genetically engineered and are available as therapeutic agents. Growth factors such as G-CSF and GM-CSF not only influence haemopoiesis but also enhance the function of the mature cells.

The details of the steady-state regulation of blood cells other than red cells are still not entirely clear. The rate of erythropoiesis is primarily regulated by the hormone erythropoietin which is secreted by the kidneys. The production of erythropoietin is stimulated when the supply of oxygen to renal tissue falls (e.g. when the red cell count falls). Erythropoietin increases red-cell production mainly by stimulating the rate of conversion of CFU-E to pronormoblasts. It also shortens the total

B-CELL DIFFERENTIATION

Characteristic	Early pre-B cell	Pre-B cell	Immature B cell	Mature B cell	Plasma cell
Heavy chain genes rearranged	+	+	+	+	+
Light chain genes rearranged	−/+	+	+	+	+
Terminal deoxynucleotidyl-transferase	+	+/−	−	−	−
Cytoplasmic μ-chains expressed	−	+	−	−	−
Surface IgM (but not IgD) expressed	−	−	+	−	−
Surface IgM and IgD expressed	−	−	−	+	−
Cytoplasmic Ig expressed	−	−	−	−	+
cALLA (CD10)	+	+	−	−	−
CD19 and CD20	+	+	+	+	+
cALLA, common acute lymphoblastic leukaemia antigen.					

Table 1.4 Sequence of events during B-cell differentiation.

T-CELL DIFFERENTIATION

Characteristic	Pre-T cell	Early thymocyte	Intermediate thymocyte	Late thymocyte	Mature T-cell
CD7	+	+	+	+	+
Terminal deoxynucleotidyl-transferase	−/+	+	+	−	−
TCR γ genes rearranged/deleted	−	+	+	+	+
TCR β genes rearranged	−	−	+	+	+
TCR α genes rearranged	−	−	−/+	+	+
CD2	−	+	+	+	+
CD3	−	+	+	+	+
CD4 and CD8	−	−	−/+	−	−
CD4 or CD8	−	−	−	+	+
TCR, T-cell receptor.					

Table 1.5 Sequence of events during T-cell differentiation.

time taken for a pronormoblast to mature into marrow reticulocytes and for the latter to be released into the circulation.

Intrauterine haemopoiesis and postnatal changes

The production of blood cells begins in the yolk sac of the 14–19 day human embryo. The fetal liver becomes the main site of haemopoiesis in the second trimester of pregnancy and the fetal bone marrow in the third trimester. The majority of the haemopoietic cells in the yolk sac and fetal liver are erythroblasts. The embryonic Hbs Gower I ($\zeta_2\varepsilon_2$), Gower II ($\alpha_2\varepsilon_2$) and Portland I ($\zeta_2\gamma_2$) are synthesized by erythroblasts in the yolk sac, fetal Hb (HbF, $\alpha_2\gamma_2$) by erythroblasts in the fetal liver, and both HbF and HbA ($\alpha_2\beta_2$) by those in the fetal bone marrow. The main site of granulocytopoietic activity in intrauterine life is the fetal bone marrow.

After birth, the marrow is the sole site of haemopoiesis in healthy individuals. During the first 4 years of life, nearly all the marrow cavities contain red haemopoietic marrow with very few fat cells. Thereafter, increasing numbers of fat cells appear in certain marrow cavities. By the age of 25 years, the only sites of active haemopoiesis are the skull bones, ribs, sternum, scapulae, clavicles, vertebrae, pelvis, the upper half of the sacrum and the proximal ends of the shafts of the femur and humerus. All the remaining marrow cavities contain yellow fatty marrow. Even at sites of active haemopoiesis, about half the volume of the marrow normally consists of fat cells.

In a number of diseases (e.g. chronic haemolytic anaemias, megaloblastic anaemias and some leukaemias) there may be: (a) a partial or complete replacement of fat cells by haemopoietic cells in marrow cavities normally supporting haemopoiesis; (b) extension of haemopoietic marrow into marrow cavities normally containing non-haemopoietic fatty marrow (e.g. in long bones); and (c) the appearance of foci of haemopoietic tissue in the liver and spleen (extramedullary haemopoiesis).

Reviews

Bessis M. (1973) *Living Blood Cells and their Ultrastructure*. Springer-Verlag, Berlin.
Grosveld F., Dillon N., Higgs D. (1993) The regulation of human globin gene expression. In: Higgs D.R., Weatherall D.J. (eds.) *The Haemoglobinopathies*. Baillière's Clinical Haematology, International Practice and Research, Vol 6/No 1. Baillière Tindall, London.
Handin R.I., Lux S.E., Stossel T.P. (eds.) (1995) *Blood, Principles & Practice of Hematology*. J.B. Lippincott, Philadelphia.

Hardisty R.M., Weatherall D.J. (eds.) (1982) *Blood and its Disorders*, 2nd edn. Blackwell Scientific Publications, Oxford.

Huisman T.H.J. (1993) The structure and function of normal and abnormal haemoglobins. In: Higgs D.R., Weatherall D.J. (eds.) *The Haemoglobinopathies*. Baillière's Clinical Haematology, International Practice and Research, Vol 6/No 1. Baillière Tindall, London.

Lee G.R., Bithell T.C., Foerster J., Athens J.W., Lukens J.N. (1993) *Wintrobe's Clinical Hematology*, 9th edn, Vols 1 & 2. Lea & Febiger, Philadelphia.

Lord B.I., Dexter T.M. (eds.) (1992) *Growth Factors in Haemopoiesis*. Baillière's Clinical Haematology, International Practice and Research, Vol 5/No 3. Baillière Tindall, London.

Nathan D.G. (ed.) (1991) The molecular biology of hematopoiesis. *Semin. Hematol.* **28**, 114–176.

Wickramasinghe S.N. (1975) *Human Bone Marrow*. Blackwell Scientific Publications, Oxford.

Wickramasinghe S.N. (1992) Bone marrow. In: Sternberg S.S. (ed.) *Histology for Pathologists*, pp. 1–31. Raven Press, New York.

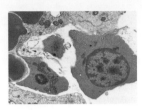

CHAPTER 2

Anaemia and Polycythaemia: General Considerations

Objectives in learning

1 To know how the symptoms and signs of anaemia and polycythaemia are caused.
2 To understand the mechanisms of production of anaemia.
3 To understand the morphological classification and diagnostic approaches to anaemia.
4 To know the causes of true and apparent polycythaemia.

Anaemia

Anaemia is said to be present when the haemoglobin (Hb) concentration is below the reference range (reference interval) for the age and sex of an individual. Reference ranges are derived from the statistical analysis of data from a sample of reference individuals, i.e. individuals selected on the basis of defined criteria. Reference ranges for Hb concentration are given in Table 2.1 These may be determined from a representative sample of healthy persons in whom the presence of iron deficiency has been excluded by specific laboratory investigations or by the prior administration of iron. In populations with a high prevalence of α- and β-thalassaemia genes, heterozygosity for thalassaemia may also have to be excluded. The average Hb level is 17.0 g/dl at birth and rises to 19.5 g/dl after 24 hours. Hb levels in children between 6 months and 6 years tend to be lower than in adults. The higher Hb levels in adult males than in adult non-pregnant females are largely due to the effects of higher androgen levels in males; the Hb levels of males fall after the age of 70 years. Hb levels are increased by residence at high altitude. Hb levels decrease during normal pregnancy, reaching their lowest value at about 32 weeks; the average fall is 1.5–2.0 g/dl. The drop in Hb concentration occurs despite an average increase in red cell mass of 300 ml, and results from an average increase in the plasma volume of about 1 litre. The Hb level may drop by 6–8% after about half an hour of bed rest.

Although reference ranges are invaluable in the assessment of a

REFERENCE RANGES	
	Hb concentration (g/dl)
Cord blood	13.5–20.5
First day of life	15.0–23.5
Children, 6 months–6 years	11.0–14.5
Children, 6–14 years	12.0–15.5
Adult males	13.0–17.0
Adult females (non-pregnant)	12.0–15.5
Pregnant females	11.0–14.0

Table 2.1 Reference ranges for Hb values.

patient, it must be realized that they do have some limitations. Thus, since reference ranges represent 95% reference limits determined on a healthy population, it would be expected that 2.5% of healthy individuals have Hb values below and 2.5% above the reference range. Therefore, not all individuals with Hb levels slightly outside the reference range would necessarily have some haematological problem. Furthermore, as the difference between the upper and lower limits of the reference range is more than 3.0 g/dl, an individual's Hb level may remain within the reference range even though it has fallen substantially due to some illness. In other words, a 'normal' Hb concentration does not necessarily exclude impairment of erythropoiesis. It also does not exclude a moderate reduction in red-cell life-span as the healthy bone marrow has a considerable physiological reserve and can increase the rate of effective erythropoiesis to six to eight times the basal rate. In patients with both anaemia and a decrease in the plasma volume secondary to dehydration, the Hb level may be spuriously high.

In healthy individuals, there are strong correlations between the Hb, red-cell count and packed cell volume (PCV). The reference ranges for the red-cell count in adult males and females are, respectively, $4.4–5.8 \times 10^{12}/l$ and $4.1–5.2 \times 10^{12}/l$. The reference ranges for the PCV in adult males and females are $0.40–0.51$ and $0.36–0.46$, respectively.

ADAPTIVE RESPONSES TO ANAEMIA

An important compensatory mechanism in anaemia consists of an increased production of 2,3-diphosphoglycerate (2,3-DPG) by red cells. This causes a reduction in the O_2 affinity of Hb (a shift of the O_2 dissociation curve to the right) and, consequently, increased release of

O_2 at tissues (p. 2). When the Hb falls below 7–8 g/dl, adaptive changes also occur in the cardiovascular system: these include an increase of cardiac output at rest mainly by an increase in stroke volume, but also by an increase in heart rate.

SYMPTOMS AND SIGNS OF ANAEMIA

Anaemia is a manifestation of disease, not a final diagnosis. The symptoms found in an anaemic patient may be caused by the underlying disease or by the anaemia itself. When anaemia develops slowly in children and young adults the symptoms referable to the anaemia are mild until the Hb falls below 7–8 g/dl. Significant symptoms develop at higher Hb levels in rapidly developing anaemias and in older patients with impaired cardiovascular reserve. Older patients are also more likely to develop cardiac and cerebral symptoms than younger ones, due to associated degenerative vascular disease.

The two mechanisms underlying the many symptoms and signs of anaemia are:

I decreased tissue oxygenation causing widespread organ dysfunction, and

2 adaptive changes, particularly in the cardiovascular system.

Symptoms include lassitude, easy fatiguability, dyspnoea on exertion, palpitation, angina and intermittent claudication (in older patients with degenerative arterial disease), headache, vertigo, light-headedness, visual disturbances, drowsiness, anorexia, nausea, bowel disturbances, menstrual disturbances, and loss of libido (see p. 83). Physical signs include pallor, tachycardia, wide pulse pressure with capillary pulsation, haemic murmurs, signs of congestive cardiac failure, and haemorrhages and occasional exudates in the retina. Severe anaemia may also cause slight proteinuria, mild impairment of renal function and low-grade fever.

MECHANISMS OF ANAEMIA

In healthy adults, there is a steady-state equilibrium between the rate of release of new red cells from the bone marrow into the circulation and the rate of removal of senescent red cells from the circulation by macrophages. The various mechanisms which may lead to anaemia are shown in Table 2.2. More than one of these mechanisms operate simultaneously in most conditions, and mechanistic classifications of the anaemias have to be based on the mechanism of greatest pathophysiological importance. Impaired red-cell formation may be due to insufficient erythropoiesis (reduced quantity of erythropoietic tissue) or to ineffective erythropoiesis (a high death rate affecting the red-cell precursors within the marrow).

MECHANISMS OF ANAEMIA

Blood loss

Decreased red-cell life-span (haemolytic anaemia)
Congenital defect (e.g. sickle-cell disease, hereditary spherocytosis)
Acquired defect (e.g. malaria, some drugs)

Impairment of red-cell formation
Insufficient erythropoiesis
Ineffective erythropoiesis

Pooling and destruction of red cells in an enlarged spleen

Increased plasma volume (splenomegaly, pregnancy)

Table 2.2 Various mechanisms leading to anaemia.

The absolute reticulocyte count (i.e. the number of reticulocytes per litre of blood) is a useful parameter with which anaemias due to increased red-cell destruction can be distinguished from those due to impaired red-cell production. This count is a relatively easily determined index of the rate of delivery of red cells into the circulation (i.e. of effective erythropoiesis). The absolute reticulocyte count (pp. 41 and 263) is increased in haemolytic anaemias as well as after acute blood loss and after treatment of iron, vitamin B_{12} or folate deficient patients with the appropriate haematinic. Reticulocyte counts are low or normal when anaemia is due to impaired red-cell production.

Blood loss

The loss of 500 ml of blood over a few minutes usually has negligible effects on the circulatory system: there is a slight fall in central venous pressure and no significant change in blood pressure or pulse rate. The rapid loss of 750 ml causes a substantial fall in central venous pressure, a fall in cardiac output and blood pressure and peripheral vasoconstriction. The acute loss of 1.5–2.0 litres of blood causes marked circulatory disturbances: the subjects are cold, clammy and restless and may become unconscious.

Immediately after an acute haemorrhage, the Hb level is normal. The acute reduction in blood volume is corrected by a slow expansion of the plasma volume over the next 36–72 hours. This results in the gradual development of a normochromic normocytic anaemia, with the lowest Hb values between 36 and 72 hours. Other changes seen in the blood after acute haemorrhage include:

1 reticulocytosis (with a peak at 7–10 days);
2 moderate neutrophil leucocytosis and mild thrombocytosis lasting for several days, and
3 the presence of metamyelocytes and occasional myelocytes in the blood film. Normoblasts may appear in the blood after severe haemorrhage.
Chronic blood loss eventually causes a hypochromic microcytic anaemia due to iron deficiency.

Other mechanisms

The anaemias resulting partly or wholly from a substantial reduction of red-cell life-span are discussed in Chapter 3. The diseases associated with impaired red-cell formation are listed in Table 2.3. In chronic renal failure, anaemia is mainly caused by decreased erythropoietin production in the diseased kidneys. Anaemia develops in endocrine deficiency syndromes because normal erythropoiesis, which is dependent on the erythroid-lineage-specific hormone erythropoietin, is also influenced by some secretions of the endocrine glands, particularly androgens and thyroxine.

IMPAIRED RED-CELL FORMATION

Deficiency of essential haematinics
Iron, folate, vitamin B_{12}, protein (see Chapters 5 and 6)

Chronic disorders (p. 90)
Infection, renal disease, liver disease, collagen disease

Marrow infiltration
Carcinoma, myeloma, leukaemia, lymphoma, myelofibrosis, lysosomal storage diseases (e.g. Gaucher's disease), marble bone disease

Endocrine deficiency
Hypofunction of the thyroid (p. 121), testes, or anterior lobe of the pituitary gland

Myelotoxic agents, aplastic anaemia and pure red-cell aplasia

Miscellaneous
Vitamin B_{12}-independent and folate-independent megaloblastic anaemias, β-thalassaemia syndromes, myelodysplastic syndromes (including primary acquired sideroblastic anaemia), congenital dyserythropoietic anaemias, malaria

Table 2.3 Causes of anaemia due to impaired red-cell formation.

MORPHOLOGICAL CLASSIFICATION OF ANAEMIA

A useful method for classifying anaemias is based on the morphology of red cells in a stained blood smear. The main terms used in such a classification are normocytic, microcytic, macrocytic, normochromic and hypochromic. *Normocytes* are red cells with a normal diameter; *microcytes* and *macrocytes* are those with a reduced and increased diameter, respectively (Fig. 2.1a–c). *Normochromia* implies normal staining of the cell, with the central area of pallor occupying about a third of the cell diameter (Fig. 2.1a) and *hypochromia* indicates reduced staining, with an increase in the central area of pallor (Fig. 2.lb). Today, morphological classification is based not only on morphological criteria but also on mean cell volumes (MCV) determined by automated blood-counting machines. It must be appreciated, however, that when blood contains only a small proportion of microcytes or macrocytes, the MCV is within the normal range. The three morphological types of anaemia and examples of conditions causing them are given in Table 2.4. The normal values for the MCV and other red-cell indices in adults are given in Table 2.5.

There are a number of morphological abnormalities of red cells other than those mentioned above which may be seen on a stained blood film in a patient with anaemia; some of these are mentioned below.

Anisocytosis and poikilocytosis

An increased degree of variation in cell diameter (anisocytosis) or cell shape (poikilocytosis) may be seen in many conditions associated with disturbed erythropoiesis. They are not specific for any disease.

Target cells

These are abnormal red cells which have a well-stained area in their middle and periphery and a pale area in between (Fig. 2.le); this appearance results from the presence of excess cell membrane relative to the volume of the cytoplasm. Target cells are found in thalassaemia syndromes, iron deficiency, sickle-cell anaemia, heterozygotes and homozygotes for HbC, homozygotes for HbE, liver disease, obstructive jaundice, hyposplenism and splenectomized individuals.

Spherocytes or microspherocytes

In several different types of haemolytic anaemia, some red cells lose their biconcave shape and become more or less spherical. In blood films, they appear as deeply stained cells which have lost their central area of pallor and which have smaller diameters than normal cells (Fig. 2.ld).

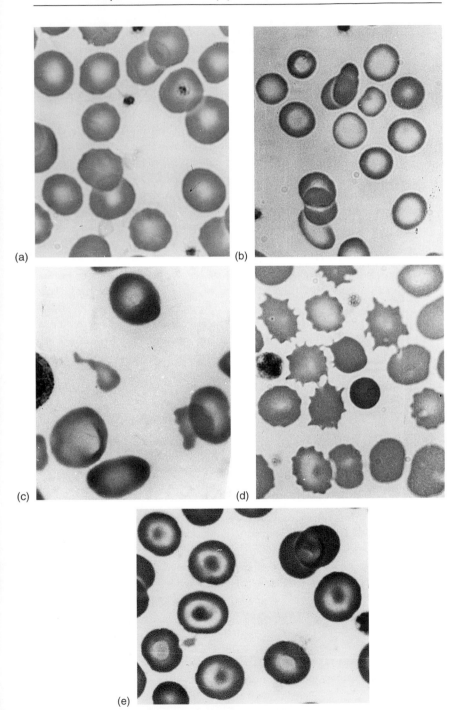

(a)

(b)

(c)

(d)

(e)

ANAEMIA: MORPHOLOGICAL TYPES

Type	MCV	Causes
Microcytic and hypochromic, or microcytic*	Low	Iron deficiency, thalassaemia syndromes, some cases of anaemia of chronic disorders
Normocytic and normochromic	Normal	Acute blood loss, some cases of anaemia of chronic disorders, some haemolytic anaemias, leucoerythroblastic anaemias
Macrocytic	High	Alcoholism, folate deficiency, vitamin B_{12} deficiency (see Chapter 6 for other causes)

MCV, mean cell volume.
*Microcytic red cells do not always appear hypochromic on a blood film.

Table 2.4 Morphological classification of anaemia.

REFERENCE RANGES

Index	Normal range
Mean cell volume* (MCV)	82–99 fl
Mean cell Hb (MCH)	27–33 pg
Mean cell Hb concentration (MCHC)	32–36 g/dl

*Lower limit may be as low as 70–74 fl between 1 and 8 years of age, in the absence of iron deficiency.

Table 2.5 Reference ranges for red-cell indices in adults.

Fig. 2.1 Normal and abnormal red cells. (a) Normochromic, normocytic cells. (b) Hypochromic microcytic cells. (c) Macrocytes and two poikilocytes. (d) One spherocyte and several acanthocytes in a blood film from a splenectomized patient. Acanthocytes are red cells with up to about ten spicules of varying length irregularly distributed over their surface. They are found not only post-splenectomy but also in other conditions such as hypothyroidism and advanced alcohol-related cirrhosis of the liver. (e) Target cells from a patient with obstructive jaundice.

Spherocytes have a reduced surface/volume ratio and usually result from:

1   an inherited abnormality of the red-cell membrane cytoskeleton (hereditary spherocytosis);

2   an acquired abnormality of the red-cell membrane (e.g. damage by clostridial toxin, or by heat, as in patients with burns);

3   ingestion of part of an antibody-coated red cell by a macrophage as in autoimmune haemolytic anaemias with warm-reactive antibodies, or

4   loss of fragments from circulating red cells by their mechanical interaction with fibrin strands or diseased vessel walls as in micro-angiopathic haemolytic anaemia.

Howell–Jolly bodies (Fig. 2.2)

These small rounded intraerythrocytic inclusions consist of nuclear material. They are found in circulating red cells following splenectomy or in patients with hyposplenism. Howell–Jolly bodies are normally present in some red cells when they leave the marrow but are rapidly removed by the spleen, possibly during the first passage of the inclusion-containing cells through that organ. Consequently, they are not found in blood films of individuals with a functioning spleen. In megaloblastic anaemias the formation of Howell–Jolly bodies within the erythroblasts in the marrow is greatly increased, and when megaloblastic haemopoiesis is associated with splenectomy or hyposplenism, the peripheral blood contains very large numbers of red cells with these inclusions.

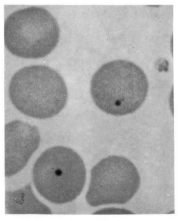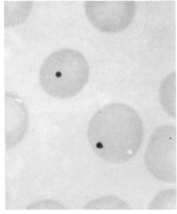

Fig. 2.2 Peripheral blood smear from a splenectomized patient with hereditary spherocytosis showing Howell–Jolly bodies within four of the red cells.

Polycythaemia (erythrocytosis)

The term 'polycythaemia' is usually applied when the packed cell volume (PCV) is repeatedly greater than 0.52 in adult males and 0.47 in adult females in peripheral blood samples taken without venous occlusion. The increase in PCV is associated with a high Hb level and a high red-cell count. Polycythaemia may result either from an increase in the total volume of red cells in the circulation (true polycythaemia) or from a decrease in the total plasma volume (apparent or relative polycythaemia). Thus, measurements of total red-cell volume (using ^{51}Cr- or ^{99m}Tc-labelled red cells) and plasma volume (using ^{125}I-albumin) are often required in the investigation of patients. The total red-cell volume (red-cell mass) is expressed as a percentage of the value predicted for the height and weight of the individual being studied; the predicted value is obtained using formulae which take some account of the amounts of relatively avascular fatty tissue in the body. A patient is considered to have true polycythaemia when the measured total red-cell volume exceeds the predicted value by more than 25% in males and 30% in females. The disorders associated with true and apparent polycythaemia are given in Table 2.6.

TRUE POLYCYTHAEMIA

An important cause of true polycythaemia, namely polycythaemia rubra vera, is discussed on p. 162. In most of the conditions listed as causing true polycythaemia due to inappropriate erythropoietin production in Table 2.6, the increased amounts of erythropoietin are either secreted by tumour cells or by compressed and hypoxic normal renal tissue surrounding renal cysts or tumours. Occasionally, there may be increased production of erythropoietin in the absence of generalized hypoxia due to an impairment of renal blood flow causing selective renal hypoxia. From the many causes of secondary polycythaemia shown, it is evident that diagnosis of the cause of a true polycythaemia may require a number of investigations, such as the measurement of the O_2 saturation of arterial blood, Hb electrophoresis (which detects two-thirds of the abnormal Hbs with a high O_2 affinity), determination of Hb–O_2 dissociation curves, intravenous pyelography, and measurement of serum erythropoietin levels.

True polycythaemia due to any cause is accompanied by an increase in whole blood viscosity. When symptoms are present, they generally result from a decrease in blood flow through the limbs, heart and brain as a consequence of the increased viscosity. In polycythaemia rubra vera, there is a high incidence of vaso-occlusive episodes related partly to the

CLASSIFICATION OF POLYCYTHAEMIA

True polycythaemia	Apparent polycythaemia (relative polycythaemia)
PRIMARY Polycythaemia rubra vera (p. 162) Idiopathic erythrocytosis (p. 166) SECONDARY *Due to generalized tissue hypoxia causing appropriately increased erythropoietin production* High altitude, cyanotic heart disease, chronic hypoxic pulmonary disease, alveolar hypoventilation due to gross obesity, heavy smoking (formation of carboxyhaemoglobin), abnormal Hbs with high O_2 affinity (e.g. Hb Chesapeake) *Due to inappropriately increased erythropoietin production* Kidney disease (carcinoma, cysts, hydronephrosis), renal transplantation, hepatocellular carcinoma, cerebellar haemangioblastoma, massive uterine fibromyomatomas	*Dehydration or plasma loss* Vomiting Diarrhoea Inadequate fluid intake Burns *Heavy smoking* *Chronic apparent polycythaemia* (Also called stress polycythaemia or Gaisböck's syndrome)

Table 2.6 Causes of true and apparent polycythaemia.

hyperviscosity and partly to a high platelet count. The risk of vaso-occlusive episodes in secondary polycythaemia has not yet been adequately documented and may be less than in polycythaemia rubra vera. However, thrombotic episodes are encountered in patients with polycythaemia secondary to cyanotic congential heart disease and occasionally in patients with high-affinity Hbs.

Whereas venesection has a clear role in the management of polycythaemia rubra vera (p. 166), its role in the management of secondary polycythaemia is less clear-cut since, in this situation, the increased red-cell mass is an adaptation to lowered arterial O_2 saturation. In considering the possible value of venesection, the advantage of the decreased viscosity and consequent increased tissue perfusion has to be balanced against the disadvantage from a decreased O_2 carrying capacity. In cyanotic congenital heart disease, some physicians cautiously venesect only those patients with symptoms attributable to hyperviscosity, bringing their PCV down to about 0.55; others cautiously venesect all patients with a PCV of 0.60 or above down to about 0.55. In polycythaemia secondary to chronic airways obstruction, venesection down to a PCV of

0.50–0.52 (but not lower) has been shown to improve cardiac function and cerebral blood flow.

APPARENT POLYCYTHAEMIA

This is commonly found as a temporary phenomenon when fluid balance is disturbed, with fluid loss exceeding fluid intake (Table 2.6).

Chronic apparent polycythaemia (spurious or stress polycythaemia) is a condition which has been reported especially in middle-aged men who are often anxious, hypertensive and obese. It is frequently associated with excessive alcohol consumption, low-dose diuretic therapy and smoking and may not be a single clinical entity. The PCV is raised but the red-cell mass is normal. This group includes some normal individuals with a red-cell mass at the upper limit of normal and a plasma volume at the lower limit of normal. In about 20% of cases, the plasma volume is reduced, sometimes to a marked degree.

Reviews

Handin R.I., Lux S.E., Stossel T.P. (eds.) (1995) *Blood. Principles & Practice of Hematology.* J.B. Lippincott, Philadelphia.

Lee G.R., Bithell T.C., Foerster J., Athens J.W., Lukens J.N. (1993) *Wintrobe's Clinical Hematology*, 9th edn, Vols 1 & 2. Lea & Febiger, Philadelphia.

Pearson T.C. (1991) Apparent polycythaemia. *Blood Rev.* **5**, 205–213.

Souid A.K., Dubansky A.S., Richman P., Sadowitz P.D. (1993) Polycythemia: a review article and case report of erythrocytosis secondary to Wilm's tumor. *Pediatr. Hematol. Oncol.* **10**, 215–221.

Territo M.C., Rosove M.H. (1991) Cyanotic congenital heart disease: hematologic management. *J. Am. Coll. Cardiol.* **18**, 320–322.

CHAPTER 3

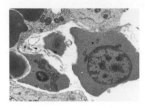

Haemolytic Anaemias

Objectives in learning

1 To know the tests for recognizing:
   (a) that red cells are being destroyed at an excessive rate, and
   (b) that the marrow is producing cells at a rate in excess of normal.

2 To know the division of haemolytic anaemias into congenital and acquired, and to know the aetiological factors in each division.

3 To understand the mode of inheritance, biochemical basis and clinical and laboratory features of hereditary spherocytosis.

4 To understand the role of glucose-6-phosphate dehydrogenase in glucose metabolism and the pathogenesis and clinical characteristics of the haemolytic syndromes which may be associated with a deficiency of this enzyme.

5 To understand the ways in which abnormalities in the structure and rate of synthesis of globin chains cause clinical and haematological abnormalities.

6 To know the clinical and laboratory manifestations of sickle-cell anaemia and the common thalassaemia syndromes; to have a general understanding of the ethnic groups in which such abnormalities are likely to occur.

7 To understand the role of autoantibodies in the production of haemolytic anaemias and to know the types of disease with which they are associated.

8 To know some of the causes of non-immune acquired haemolytic anaemias.

The haemolytic anaemias are a group of diseases in which red-cell life-span is shortened. It should be noted that a patient with a diminished red-cell life-span is not always anaemic. When the rate of red-cell destruction is increased, red-cell production in the marrow is stimulated through the erythropoietin mechanism in an attempt to maintain the haemoglobin (Hb) concentration at the normal level. In the majority of haemolytic anaemias, the marrow responds optimally to this stimulus and increases the red-cell output up to a maximum of six to eight times normal. Thus, when patients have only a moderately reduced red-cell life-span, say 20–30 days instead of the normal 120 days, they increase the rate of red-cell production sufficiently to maintain the Hb concentration within normal limits, provided that their Hb does not give up O_2 more readily than normal and their bone marrow is healthy. Such individuals are described as having a compensated haemolytic state rather than a haemolytic anaemia. On the other hand, a life-span of 5–10 days, irrespective of its cause, is always associated with anaemia.

A sub-optimal marrow response is seen when there is a lack of iron, vitamin B_{12} or folic acid; when the red-cell precursors are damaged (sometimes by the agent causing the haemolysis); when the marrow is infiltrated by malignant cells (e.g. in chronic lymphocytic leukaemia complicated by an autoimmune haemolytic anaemia); and in homozygous β-thalassaemia.

In the majority of haemolytic anaemias, the macrophages in the spleen, liver and bone marrow remove the abnormal red cells from the circulation by phagocytosis (extravascular haemolysis). In a minority, the red cells rupture and release their Hb intravascularly (intravascular haemolysis).

Many conditions are associated with a haemolytic process. The most commonly encountered include hereditary spherocytosis, hereditary elliptocytosis, glucose-6-phosphate dehydrogenase deficiency, sickle-cell anaemia, thalassaemia and the acquired haemolytic anaemias.

Evidence of haemolysis

Since haemolysis is usually associated with increased erythropoiesis, two categories of laboratory evidence can be looked for in a patient suspected of suffering from a haemolytic state. These are: (a) evidence of increased red-cell destruction; and (b) evidence of a compensatory increase in erythropoietic activity (Tabbara 1992).

LABORATORY EVIDENCE OF INCREASED RED-CELL DESTRUCTION

The various types of evidence in this category are summarized in Table 3.1.

Biochemical consequences of extravascular haemolysis

The simplest method of obtaining evidence of increased red-cell destruction is by estimating the amount of unconjugated bilirubin in plasma. When the red cell is destroyed within macrophages, the haem is converted into bilirubin with the release of carbon monoxide. Unconjugated

INCREASED DESTRUCTION

Biochemical consequences of extravascular haemolysis
Hyperbilirubinaemia (unconjugated)
Reduced serum haptoglobin

Biochemical consequences of intravascular haemolysis
Reduced serum haptoglobin
Haemoglobinaemia
Haemoglobinuria
Haemosiderinuria
Methaemalbuminaemia*
Reduced haemopexin levels*

Morphological evidence of damage to red cells
Microspherocytes, red-cell fragments, sickle cells

Reduced red-cell life-span

* Now rarely used in investigating a patient.

Table 3.1 Laboratory findings indicative of increased red-cell destruction.

bilirubin is insoluble in water and hence is transported to the liver attached to albumin. In the liver it is converted into the soluble glucuronide and excreted. The healthy liver is capable of handling more bilirubin than is normally produced and is able to increase its bilirubin-handling capacity further in haemolytic states. However, there is an upper limit for the rate of glucuronide formation by the liver and when the supply of bilirubin exceeds this rate, the unconjugated bilirubin concentration in the plasma rises. Bilirubin concentration therefore does not rise above the normal range when there is only a moderate increase in the rate of destruction of red cells. It begins to rise when the life-span is shortened to about 50 days or less. A rise in plasma bilirubin concentration is only significant in the diagnosis of a haemolytic process if liver function is entirely normal.

Biochemical consequences of intravascular haemolysis

The Hb released from intravascular lysis of red cells binds to the specific Hb-binding protein in the plasma, namely haptoglobin. Since the Hb–haptoglobin complexes are rapidly taken up by hepatocytes, intravascular haemolysis leads to a reduction in haptoglobin levels. Haptoglobins are also reduced in extravascular haemolysis, due to the escape of some Hb from the macrophages when they phagocytose damaged red cells.

When the quantity of Hb released during intravascular haemolysis exceeds the Hb binding capacity of haptoglobin, free Hb is found in the plasma (haemoglobinaemia). Haem is released from the Hb and rapidly becomes oxidized to haematin. The oxidized haem initially binds to the specific haem-binding protein in plasma, haemopexin, and the haem–haemopexin complexes are cleared by hepatocytes. After the haemopexin molecules are saturated, the haematin binds to albumin to form methaemalbumin which can be detected by the Schumm's test. When haemoglobinaemia is present, some of the free Hb dissociates into dimers and the dimers pass through the glomerulus, thus causing haemoglobinuria. Some of the dimers are taken up by renal tubular cells and converted within the cells to haemosiderin. The haemosiderin may be detected in spun deposits of urine both inside shed tubular cells and extracellularly, using Perls' acid ferrocyanide reaction.

Morphological evidence of damage to red cells

A careful examination of a blood film may indicate the occurrence of haemolysis by revealing the presence of damaged or abnormal red cells such as microspherocytes, red-cell fragments (schistocytes), sickled red cells or cells containing malarial parasites.

Reduced red-cell life-span

The most direct way to show that there is increased red-cell destruction is to measure the red-cell life-span and demonstrate that it is shortened. The red cells are usually labelled with radioactive chromium (^{51}Cr) and reinjected into the patient (Mollison et al. 1987). The survival of the labelled cells is then followed by taking blood samples at intervals and measuring their radioactivity (Fig. 3.1). By placing a γ-ray detector on the surface of the body over the spleen and liver, an indication of the main site of red-cell destruction can also be obtained; when the ^{51}Cr accumulates predominantly in the spleen, splenectomy is usually followed by a partial or complete cure of the haemolytic process. Red-cell life-span measurements are rarely needed to diagnose haemolysis.

LABORATORY EVIDENCE OF INCREASED ERYTHROPOIETIC ACTIVITY

If evidence can be obtained of an increased rate of red-cell production, this suggests that a haemolytic process is taking place, providing that there has been no loss of red cells through haemorrhage and the patient is not responding to therapy with iron, vitamin B$_{12}$, or folate. Two simple measurements can be used for assessing whether there is any increase in the rate of formation of red cells, namely, the reticulocyte count in the peripheral blood and the myeloid/erythroid ratio in the marrow (Table 3.2).

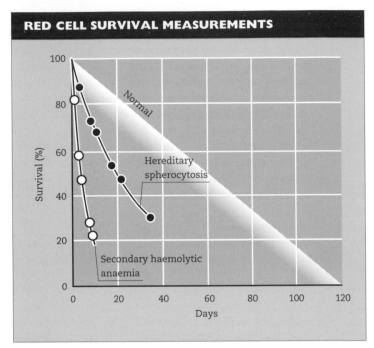

Fig. 3.1 The survival of 51Cr-labelled red cells (corrected for 51Cr elution) in the circulation of a patient with hereditary spherocytosis (●) whose Hb concentration was 15.5 g/dl, the mean red-cell life-span 30 days; a patient with autoimmune haemolytic anaemia secondary to chronic lymphocytic leukaemia (○), whose Hb concentration was 5 g/dl, the mean red-cell life-span 5 days.

INCREASED PRODUCTION

Peripheral blood
Reticulocytosis and erythroblastaemia; macrocytosis

Bone marrow
Erythroid hyperplasia; reduced myeloid/erythroid ratio

Bone
Changes in the skull and tubular bones

Table 3.2 Evidence of increased erythropoietic activity.

Reticulocytosis (increased reticulocyte count)

The number of reticulocytes in the blood is expressed either as a percentage of the total number of red cells or as an absolute number per litre of blood; in normal adults, the percentage is in the range of 0.5–3.0% and the absolute count is $20–130 \times 10^9/l$. In theory, the total number of reticulocytes in the circulation should be proportional to the rate of production of red cells, provided that there is no variation in the length of time that reticulocytes take to mature. In practice, reticulocytes released prematurely from the marrow following erythropoietin stimulation spend longer in the circulation than normal reticulocytes before they mature into adult cells. Nevertheless, an increase in the absolute reticulocyte count is an indication of increased erythropoietic activity and in general, the higher the count, the greater the rate of delivery of viable red cells to the circulation. The reticulocyte percentage may increase up to 50% or more when erythropoietic activity is intense.

Erythroblastaemia and macrocytosis

Moderate or marked erythroid hyperplasia may be associated with the presence of occasional nucleated red cells (erythroblasts) in the circulation (erythroblastaemia). A high mean cell volume (MCV) that is unrelated to folate deficiency may also occur. This macrocytosis is related to the presence of a high proportion of reticulocytes in the blood; the reticulocytes formed during accelerated erythropoiesis are abnormally large and mature into rounded macrocytes. In addition, chronic erythroid hyperplasia imposes an increased demand for folate and if this is not met by adequate dietary intake, macrocytosis due to folate deficiency develops.

Erythroid hyperplasia and reduced myeloid/erythroid (M/E) ratio

A semi-quantitative assessment of the degree of erythroid hyperplasia can be obtained by determining the myeloid/erythroid (M/E) ratio in the bone marrow. This is often defined as the ratio between the number of cells of the neutrophil series (including mature granulocytes) and the number of erythroblasts in bone marrow. The normal range for the M/E ratio in marrow smears from adults is two to eight (i.e. there are normally more cells of the neutrophil series than erythroblasts). A reduction of the M/E ratio is taken as evidence of erythroid hyperplasia, provided that the total number of cells of the neutrophil series can be assumed to be normal. Marrows showing erythroid hyperplasia are hypercellular, due to the replacement of fat cells by erythroblasts (Plates 11–13). When erythroid hyperplasia is marked, fat cells may be virtually absent. Also, haemopoietic tissue may extend into marrow cavities which usually contain only fat, and extramedullary haemopoiesis may develop in the liver, spleen and lymph nodes.

Erythroid hyperplasia occurs not only in haemolytic states and after haemorrhage but also in megaloblastic and sideroblastic anaemias (where erythropoiesis is markedly ineffective, see p. 17), polycythaemia and erythroleukaemia.

CLINICAL FEATURES OF HAEMOLYTIC STATES

These result both from the increased red-cell destruction and from the compensatory increase in erythropoietic activity. There may be pallor and mild jaundice. The prevalence of pigment stones in the gall bladder is increased; the stones may occasionally cause deep jaundice due to biliary obstruction. Splenomegaly is common. In patients with severe congenital haemolytic anaemias, the erythroid hyperplasia causes expansion of marrow cavities, thinning of cortical bone, bone deformities (e.g. frontal and

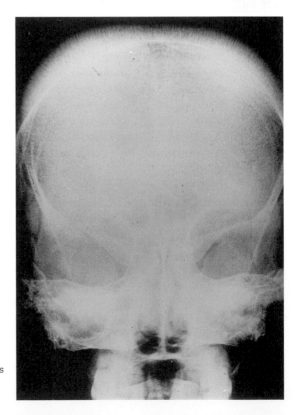

Fig. 3.2 X-ray of the skull of a patient with homozygous β-thalassaemia. The space between the abnormally thin tables of the skull bones is considerably widened due to erythroid hyperplasia. Bone trabeculae have developed at right angles to the tables giving a 'hair-on-end' appearance.

parietal bossing) and, very occasionally, pathological fractures. These changes cause characteristic radiological abnormalities in the skull and other bones (Fig. 3.2). Occasionally, chronic leg ulcers develop over the malleoli.

Aplastic crises

Episodes of pure red-cell aplasia, lasting about a week, may complicate the course of patients with chronic haemolytic anaemia. Erythroblasts virtually disappear from the marrow, the absolute reticulocyte count falls markedly (sometimes to zero) and the Hb falls rapidly. Such crises are often preceded by a febrile illness, with gastrointestinal symptoms, joint pains and, rarely, a maculopapular or erythematous rash and are usually caused by infection of erythroid progenitor cells with parvovirus B19. Affected patients may have to be transfused with red cells urgently.

Diagnosis of haemolytic anaemia

There are two stages in the diagnosis of haemolytic anaemia:
1 the demonstration of a haemolytic state, and
2 the determination of its aetiology.

The diagnosis of a haemolytic state is commonly made with reasonable confidence by the finding of an increase in both the reticulocyte count and the plasma bilirubin concentration, in a patient in whom alternative causes for these two abnormalities are excluded, e.g. haemorrhage and liver disease. Anaemia may or may not be present. Other findings indicating haemolysis have been discussed above (see Tables 3.1 and 3.2).

The next stage in diagnosis is to determine the nature of the disease which is causing the haemolysis. In approaching the diagnosis, it is useful to make a distinction between congenital abnormalities of the red cells on the one hand, and acquired abnormalities on the other. In the latter category, an agent acts on the red cell leading to its destruction, e.g. autoantibodies in autoimmune haemolytic anaemia. Congenital haemolytic anaemias may result from defects in one of three components of the red cell:
1 cell membrane;
2 enzyme systems concerned with the energy production that maintains the integrity of the cell, and
3 Hb.

Congenital haemolytic anaemias

DEFECTS OF THE RED-CELL MEMBRANE

There is a submembranous filamentous protein meshwork which is attached to the inner surface of the red-cell membrane, called the membrane cytoskeleton. The four main proteins in this cytoskeleton are spectrin, actin, protein 4.1 and ankyrin. The cytoskeleton seems to be important for maintaining the normal biconcave shape of the red cell.

Hereditary spherocytosis

The most common haemolytic anaemia due to a membrane defect is hereditary spherocytosis (HS). Recent evidence indicates that there are various types of primary molecular defects, such as mutations leading to a partial deficiency of spectrin, ankyrin, band 3 or protein 4.2 (Palek & Jarolim 1993). It has been proposed that these deficiencies lead to uncoupling of the cytoskeleton from the overlying lipid bilayer membrane and, consequently, to the release of bilayer lipids in the form of skeleton-free lipid vesicles. The loss of lipid results in a reduction of surface area and thus causes the older red cells to become microspherocytes. Repeated passage through the spleen aggravates the spherocytic change. Spherocytes are less deformable than normal red cells and are therefore retarded and eventually prevented from passing from the Billroth cords to the splenic sinusoids. The trapped cells are engulfed and destroyed by splenic macrophages, leading to a reduction in red-cell survival.

The prevalence of the disease in North Europe has been estimated to be 1 per 5000 of the population. The disease is usually inherited as an autosomal dominant character. Patients often give a family history of the condition, such as a parent or sibling who is known to have the disease or who has had recurrent anaemia, gall stones or a splenectomy.

The disease may present at any time from birth to old-age. There is a great difference in the severity of the disease, varying from patients who have an Hb concentration of 4–5 g/dl, to patients who are not anaemic at all. Mackinney (1965) investigated 26 families and found that half the patients had no symptoms but had abnormalities in the peripheral blood. He also found that half of the non-splenectomized patients had Hb concentrations of over 12 g/dl.

Apart from anaemia and jaundice, the main clinical finding in most patients is an enlarged spleen. Most patients develop pigment stones in the gall bladder and 10–20% of those with intact spleens also develop acute cholecystitis or biliary obstruction.

Trivial viral illnesses may lead to episodes of increased red-cell destruction during which the patient becomes more anaemic and jaundiced and frequently develops abdominal pain. Aplastic crises due to a temporary failure of red-cell production by the bone marrow may also occur and are usually caused by parvovirus B19 (p. 43). Patients may present for the first time during a haemolytic or aplastic episode.

Megaloblastic anaemia due to folate deficiency is also occasionally found, as in other chronic haemolytic disorders. This results from an increased requirement for folate by the hyperactive bone marrow, and is especially found when the diet is inadequate.

Diagnosis

The cardinal clinical features are a family history, mild jaundice, pallor and splenomegaly. The laboratory findings which are of the greatest help in diagnosis are: the presence of spherocytes in the stained blood-film (Fig. 3.3, Plate 45); an increased reticulocyte count; raised plasma bilirubin; increased osmotic fragility of the red cells; and a negative antiglobulin test (which excludes spherocytosis due to an autoantibody). The spherocytes appear as small densely staining cells and the percentage of spherocytes varies markedly from patient to patient. An important test which must always be carried out when spherocytes are infrequent is the osmotic fragility test. When normal red cells are suspended in a range of hypotonic saline solutions, they do not start to lyse until the saline concentration is reduced below 0.55 g/dl. In hereditary spherocytosis, the red cells are thicker than normal and some are already spherocytic, so that a smaller amount of fluid uptake than normal is sufficient to burst

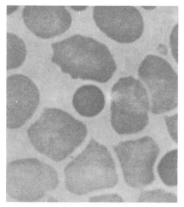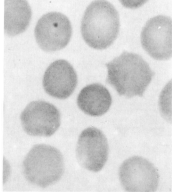

Fig. 3.3 Blood film from a patient with hereditary spherocytosis. There is one spherocyte in the centre of each photograph.

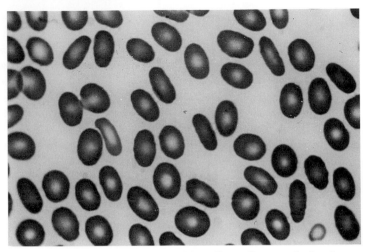

Fig. 3.4 Blood film from a patient with hereditary elliptocytosis showing a
high proportion of elliptical red cells.

the cells (i.e. the cells have an increased osmotic fragility). Thus, these
abnormal cells start to lyse when the saline concentration is as high as
0.6–0.8 g/dl.

Treatment

Severely anaemic and symptomatic moderately anaemic patients are
subjected to splenectomy. Since splenectomy, particularly in children
under the age of 5 years, is associated with an increased risk of fatal
infections, it should be delayed until after the age of 5–10 years, whenever possible. Furthermore, the risk of overwhelming infection should
be minimized by the administration of pneumococcal vaccine prior
to splenectomy, and of prophylactic Penicillin V post-splenectomy.
Splenectomy regularly results in a rise in the Hb level, the disappearance
of jaundice and an increase of red-cell life-span to almost normal values.
However, spherocytosis persists.

Hereditary elliptocytosis

This condition, which affects 1 per 2500 of the population, is transmitted
as an autosomal dominant trait. Characteristically, 25–90% of the red
cells are oval, elliptical or rod-shaped (Fig. 3.4), whereas in a blood smear
from a normal person only 0–5% of cells have this morphology. Most
heterozygotes either do not have a shortened red-cell life-span or show
evidence of a compensated haemolytic state. A few have a chronic

symptomatic haemolytic anaemia. Homozygotes usually have a severe haemolytic anaemia from infancy.

The underlying defect is an abnormality in the membrane leading to a progressive failure to restore the circular shape of the red cell following repeated elliptical deformation in the microcirculation. Patients have various mutations affecting the spectrin genes or, rarely, the protein 4.1 or glycophorin C genes, which lead to abnormalities in the association of spectrin dimers into tetramers, partial or complete deficiency of protein 4.1, a structurally abnormal protein 4.1 or absence of glycophorin C (Palek & Jarolim 1993).

ABNORMALITIES OF RED-CELL ENZYMES

Haemolytic anaemias may also result from congenital abnormalities of the enzyme system concerned with energy transfer in glucose metabolism (Mentzer 1981). The red cell requires a continuous supply of energy for the maintenance of membrane flexibility and cell shape, the regulation of sodium and potassium pumps, and the maintenance of Hb in the reduced ferrous form. The energy is obtained from glucose, which is converted to lactic acid mainly through the anaerobic glycolytic cycle (Embden–Meyerhof pathway). There is an alternative aerobic pathway, the pentose–phosphate shunt, starting with glucose-6-phosphate and requiring glucose-6-phosphate dehydrogenase (G6PD) as the initial enzyme (Fig. 3.5). Energy is transferred through the energy-rich compounds adenosine triphosphate (ATP), reduced nicotinamide-adenine dinucleotide (NADH), the related phosphorylated compound, NADPH, and reduced glutathione (GSH).

The most common enzyme deficiency giving rise to a haemolytic anaemia is deficiency of G6PD, an enzyme within the pentose–phosphate shunt. Occasionally, deficiencies of other enzymes cause a congenital non-spherocytic haemolytic anaemia, e.g. deficiency of pyruvate kinase, an enzyme within the anaerobic glycolytic pathway.

Glucose-6-phosphate dehydrogenase deficiency

There are two types of normal G6PD enzyme. The most prevalent world-wide is designated type B. About 20% of healthy Africans have type A, which has normal enzyme activity and results from a single amino acid change from type B. It has been estimated that there may be as many as a hundred million people in the world who have diminished red cell G6PD activity. The defective gene is present on the X-chromosome, and thus the clinical features of G6PD deficiency are mainly seen in males ($\overline{X}Y$, where $\overline{X}$ is the abnormal chromosome). Homozygous women ($\overline{X}\overline{X}$) are also clinically affected but such individuals are uncommon. The

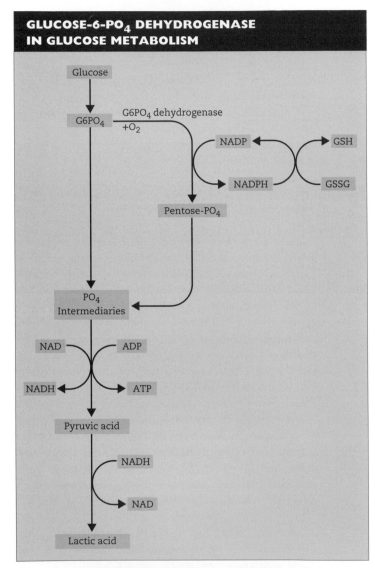

Fig. 3.5 A schematic diagram of the pathway of glucose metabolism in the red cell, to show the important role of glucose-6-phosphate dehydrogenase. Decreased activity of the enzyme leads to a deficiency of the reducing compounds NADPH and GSH.

normal X-chromosome in heterozygous women ($\overline{\text{X}}$X) usually maintains sufficient G6PD activity to prevent clinical manifestations. The high prevalence of G6PD deficiency must have some Darwinian survival value and there is evidence indicating that deficiency gives some protection to the heterozygous female against *Plasmodium falciparum*; G6PD deficiency is common only in populations exposed for long periods to tertian malaria — heterozygous females with malaria have lower parasite counts in their red cells than normal women.

Deficiency of the enzyme is found in about 20% of blacks from West Africa and, to a varying extent, in southern Europe, the Middle East, India, Thailand and southern China. Deficiency is very rare in Caucasians. Virtually all of the 400 or so known variants of G6PD arise from single point mutations within the coding region of the G6PD gene (Vulliamy *et al.* 1992). Only two variants are common and these account for over 95% of cases. The most common is the African (or A-) type, where G6PD function is reduced to about 10% of normal; in the less common Mediterranean type, the enzyme activity is reduced to 1–3%.

Low activities of G6PD result in low concentrations of the reducing compounds NADPH and GSH (see Fig. 3.5). The purpose of these compounds is to maintain Hb and other erythrocytic proteins in a reduced and active form. People with low levels of the enzymes are thus poorly protected against drugs which are oxidants. When oxidants enter the cell they first convert Hb to methaemoglobin and finally denature it so that it precipitates in the red cell in the form of rounded masses known as Heinz bodies (Plate 15). These Heinz bodies (and the portion of the red-cell membrane to which they become attached) are removed by splenic macrophages as the red cells pass through the spleen; the resulting inclusion-free cells stain densely, display unstained areas at their periphery ('bite' cells) (Plate 16) and undergo extravascular haemolysis. Components of the red-cell membrane may also undergo marked oxidation leading to intravascular haemolysis. Oxidant drugs which bring about this type of haemolytic anaemia include the anti-malarial drugs (e.g. primaquine), sulphonamides, analgesics such as aspirin (high doses) and phenacetin, and vitamin K analogues.

A number of screening tests and assays for detecting G6PD deficiency are available. These are based on assessing the production of NADPH by red cells in the presence of an excess of glucose-6-phosphate. The NADPH is detected spectrophotometrically, or by its ability to reduce nitroblue tetrazolium (NBT) in the presence of an electron transfer agent, or by its ability to fluoresce in ultraviolet light.

A variety of clinical syndromes may be associated with G6PD variants which have reduced enzyme activity. These are outlined below.

Episodic acute haemolysis
Most of the time, patients with the two common G6PD variants (A- and Mediterranean types) are symptomless and have normal Hb concentrations with only a slight shortening of the red-cell life-span. Episodes of haemolytic anaemia develop during infections or following exposure to oxidant drugs and chemicals. Anaemia is maximal about 7–10 days after taking an oxidant. The extent of the fall in Hb concentration is partly dependent on the amount and nature of the drug being given, and partly on the extent of reduction of enzyme activity. In patients with the A-variant, after about 10 days and despite continuation of the drug, the Hb concentration rises again and may reach normal levels. This is due to the fact that in these patients only the older cells have sufficiently low G6PD activities to be affected and destroyed by the drug. Heinz bodies may be demonstrated in circulating red cells during the early stages of haemolytic episodes. In patients with the Mediterranean type, in whom the average enzyme activity is very low, haemolysis may not be self-limiting.

Neonatal jaundice
Hyperbilirubinaemia, sometimes necessitating exchange transfusion, is occasionally found in G6PD-deficient neonates. The hyperbilirubinaemia may be due to hepatocyte dysfunction or oxidant damage to red cells. Affected individuals recover completely after the neonatal period but may develop episodic acute haemolysis (see above), during later life.

Congenital non-spherocytic haemolytic anaemia
Very rarely, the reduction in G6PD activity is so marked that there is substantial haemolysis and anaemia throughout life.

Favism
Favism has been known for 2000 years or more. It is an acute haemolytic anaemia occurring after the ingestion of the broad bean (*Vicia fava*) in individuals with a deficiency of G6PD (commonly of the Mediterranean type). Favism usually affects children; severe anaemia develops rapidly and is often accompanied by haemoglobinuria. Fava beans contain two β-glycosides, vicine and convicine, which generate free radicals and consequently oxidize GSH and other red-cell constituents.

ABNORMALITIES OF THE STRUCTURE OR SYNTHESIS OF HAEMOGLOBIN

Hb molecules present in fetal and postnatal life are composed of four polypeptide (globin) chains, two α- and two non-α-chains, which combine together to form a globular protein. Each globin chain is associated with a single haem group which can reversibly combine with O_2. Most of the Hb in a normal adult is called haemoglobin A (HbA) and contains two α- and two β-chains ($\alpha_2\beta_2$). Between 1.5 and 3.5% consists of haemoglobin A_2 ($\alpha_2\delta_2$) and less than 1% consists of haemoglobin F or fetal haemoglobin ($\alpha_2\gamma_2$).

Inherited abnormalities of Hb fall into two categories (Lehmann & Huntsman 1974; Weatherall & Clegg 1981; Higgs & Weatherall 1993):

1 *structural Hb variants (haemoglobinopathies)* in which there is an alteration in the amino acid sequence of a globin chain without a reduction in the rate of synthesis of the abnormal chain, and

2 *thalassaemia syndromes* in which there is a depression in the rate of synthesis of one of the globin chains.

> In the thalassaemia syndromes, the amino acid sequences of the globin chains are usually normal. However, a thalassaemic blood picture may sometimes arise from the presence of a structurally abnormal globin chain which is synthesized at a reduced rate (e.g. Hb Constant Spring and Hb Lepore) or of an abnormal Hb which is markedly unstable (e.g. Hb Indianapolis).

STRUCTURAL HAEMOGLOBIN VARIANTS

Over 600 abnormal Hbs have been reported but most are rare and only a few lead to clinical or haematological manifestations. The majority of structural Hb variants are the consequence of a single-point mutation affecting one base triplet (codon) in a globin gene and, therefore, have a single amino acid substitution in the affected globin chain (e.g. HbS, HbE, HbC and HbD).

> If a single-point mutation affects the stop codon of the α-globin gene, the α-chains produced have extra amino acids at one end (e.g. in Hb Constant Spring). A few abnormal Hbs result from deletions of one or more base triplets or insertions of extra base triplets, consequently showing a loss of one or more amino acids or a gain of amino acids within a chain, respectively. An occasional variant results from fusion genes and contains hybrid chains made of parts of δ- and β-chains (in Hb Lepore) or γ- and β-chains (in Hb Kenya).

The spectrum of clinical and haematological abnormalities that may be caused by abnormal Hbs is summarized in Table 3.3. The most common structural Hb variant is haemoglobin S (HbS) and this is discussed in some detail below.

When the amino acid substitution results in an overall change in the charge of the molecule, its migration in a voltage gradient is altered

EFFECTS OF HAEMOGLOBIN VARIANTS

Variant	Clinical and haematological abnormalities
HbS	Recurrent painful crises (in adults) and chronic haemolytic anaemia; both related to sickling of red cells on deoxygenation*
HbC	Chronic haemolytic anaemia due to reduced red-cell deformability on deoxygenation*; deoxygenated HbC is less soluble than deoxygenated HbA
Hb Köln, Hb Hammersmith	Spontaneous or drug-induced haemolytic anaemia due to instability of the Hb and consequent intracellular precipitation
HbM Boston or HbM Saskatoon	Cyanosis due to congenital methaemoglobinaemia as a consequence of a substitution near or in the haem-pocket
Hb Chesapeake	Hereditary polycythaemia due to increased O_2 affinity
Hb Kansas	Anaemia and cyanosis due to decreased O_2 affinity
Hb Constant Spring, Hb Lepore, HbE	Thalassaemia-like syndrome due to decreased rate of synthesis of abnormal chain
Hb Indianapolis	Thalassaemia-like syndrome due to marked instability of Hb

* Only in homozygotes.

Table 3.3 Different clinical and haematological abnormalities associated with some structural haemoglobin variants.

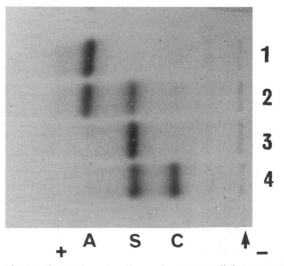

Fig. 3.6 Electrophoresis of haemolysates on cellulose acetate (pH 8.5). The arrow marks the site of application of the haemolysate. (1) Normal adult. (2) Individual with sickle-cell trait; 35% of the Hb consists of HbS and most of the remainder is HbA. (3) Patient with sickle-cell anaemia: most of the Hb is S and there is no A. (4) Double heterozygote for HbS and HbC. This results in a disease which is usually milder than that in homozygotes for HbS.

and this can be demonstrated by standard electrophoretic techniques. The speed of migration is characteristic for each abnormal Hb (Fig. 3.6).

Haemoglobin S

In this Hb, the charged glutamic acid residue in position 6 of the normal β-chain is replaced by an uncharged valine molecule. This results in deoxygenated HbS being 50 times less soluble than deoxygenated HbA. The deoxygenated HbS molecules initially polymerize without forming fibres and subsequently polymerize into long fibres (tactoids) (Fig. 3.7) which deform the red cell into the typical sickle-shape (Fig. 3.8). Red cells from heterozygotes for HbS sickle at much lower Po_2 values than those from homozygotes, and do not usually sickle *in vivo*.

The gene for HbS occurs especially in a wide area across tropical

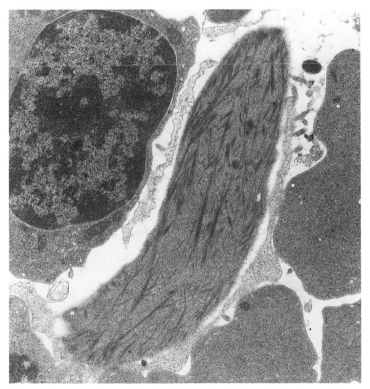

Fig. 3.7 Electron micrograph of a sickled red cell from a homozygote for HbS showing fibres of polymerized deoxygenated HbS running along the long axis of the cell.

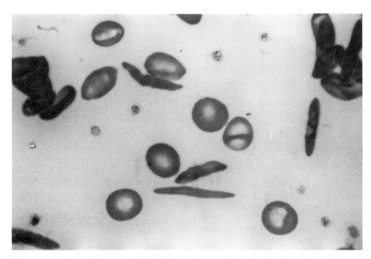

Fig. 3.8 Four sickle cells (with pointed ends) from the blood film of a patient with sickle-cell anaemia (homozygote for HbS).

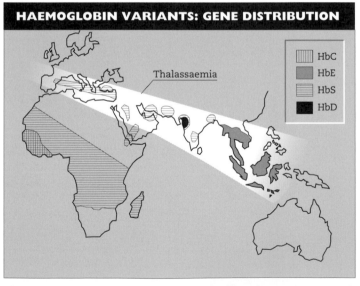

Fig. 3.9 Distribution of the genes for the major Hb variants – S, E, C, D and thalassaemia.

Africa, in some countries bordering on the northern shores of the Mediterranean, and in parts of the Middle East and southern India (Fig. 3.9). The prevalence of this gene in these areas varies from very low values to 40% of the population. In black Americans, the prevalence is 8%. The distribution of the HbS gene corresponds to areas in which falciparum malaria has been endemic; the persistence of this potentially lethal gene in high frequency in these areas results from the fact that heterozygotes die less frequently from severe falciparum malaria during early childhood than children with only HbA.

Sickle-cell trait

Heterozygotes (one gene for HbA and one for HbS) are described as having sickle-cell trait. Their red cells contain between 20 and 45% HbS, the rest being mainly HbA. Heterozygotes do not have 50% HbS mainly because mutant β-chains (β^s) have a lower affinity than normal β-chains to associate with α-chains. Individuals with sickle-cell trait are haematologically normal and are usually asymptomatic. However, spontaneous haematuria may occur occasionally and renal papillary necrosis rarely. Furthermore, there is often an impaired ability to concentrate urine in older individuals. The red cells do not sickle in the trait until the O_2 saturation falls below 40%, a level which is rarely reached in venous blood. Painful crises (see p. 57) and splenic infarction have occurred in severely hypoxic individuals.

Sickle-cell anaemia

Homozygotes for HbS are described as having sickle-cell anaemia. Their red cells contain 80% or more HbS, the remainder being mainly fetal Hb. The cells sickle at the O_2 tension normally found in venous blood. Initially, there are cycles of sickling and reversal of sickling as the red cells are repeatedly deoxygenated and oxygenated within the circulation. Eventually, irreversibly sickled cells are formed. Both unsickled and sickled red cells containing deoxygenated HbS are less deformable than normal red cells and suffer mainly extravascular haemolysis. The increased rigidity of the cells may cause them to become jammed in and obstruct small and, occasionally, medium-sized blood vessels, thus causing tissue infarction. Symptoms due to infarction are not present continuously but occur in episodes.

There is a chronic haemolytic anaemia at all ages, with the Hb usually varying between 6 and 9 g/dl; the symptoms of anaemia are milder than expected from the Hb levels as HbS has a reduced affinity for O_2 (O_2 dissociation curve shifted to the right) (p. 2). The haemolysis may lead to the formation of pigment gallstones. Different tissues are liable to

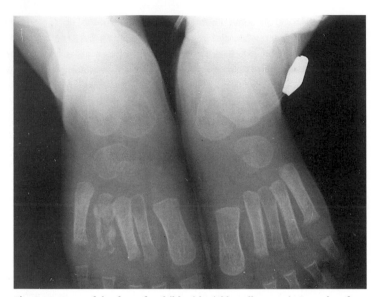

Fig. 3.10 X-ray of the feet of a child with sickle-cell anaemia 2 weeks after the onset of the hand–foot syndrome, showing necrosis of the right fourth metatarsal.

infarction at different ages so that the clinical picture varies markedly with age (Sergeant 1985; Higgs & Weatherall 1993). Furthermore, some patients are only mildly affected having few or no infarctive episodes at any age. In some of these patients, the mildness of the disease is related to the co-inheritance of one or two α-thalassaemia genes (which reduces the mean cell Hb concentration (MCHC)) or a gene for the hereditary persistence of HbF.

A characteristic feature of sickle-cell anaemia in infancy and early childhood is dactylitis, or the hand–foot syndrome, resulting from occlusion of the nutrient arteries to the metacarpals and metatarsals (Fig. 3.10). There is a painful, non-erythematous and often symmetrical swelling of the hands and feet, lasting 10–14 days. Infants and young children may also develop a life threatening splenic sequestration syndrome. Here there is rapid and extensive trapping of red cells in the spleen leading to profound anaemia, massive splenomegaly, reduced blood volume and hypovolaemic shock. Sickle-cell anaemia patients show an increased susceptibility to fulminant bacterial infections, especially in the first 3 years of life, apparently due to a combination of hyposplenism (despite the splenomegaly) and an abnormality in opsonization.

The acute chest syndrome (acute febrile illness with dyspnoea, chest pain and radiological changes) is the most common cause of death after the age of 2 years; this syndrome results from a combination of pulmonary infection, infarction and sequestration. Strokes due to cerebral infarction may also occur, especially between the ages of three and ten.

In older children and adults, recurrent episodes of widespread microvascular occlusion lead to painful crises. These usually consist of attacks of pain affecting the bones and large joints of all four limbs and the back. The crises are accompanied by low-grade fever and may last from a few days to a few weeks. Occasionally the pain may be felt predominantly in one limb or in the chest or abdomen. Patients in this age-group also suffer from larger infarcts affecting the bones (leading to avascular necrosis of the heads of the femora or humeri and of the diaphyses of long bones). The spleen is usually palpable in children, but it atrophies from repeated infarction and is usually not felt in adults.

Other clinical features include *Salmonella* infection of necrotic bone (osteomyelitis), chronic leg ulcers (Fig. 3.11) and priapism. Some patients develop chronic pulmonary disease or cor pulmonale. Almost all the patients show abnormalities of retinal vessels on ophthalmoscopy. Aplastic crises due to parvovirus infection may occur (p. 43) as may an aggravation of the anaemia due to a secondary folate deficiency (p. 41). Patients are unable to concentrate urine normally from an early age. Occasionally, painless haematuria develops due to small medullary infarcts or papillary necrosis. The nephrotic syndrome may develop in

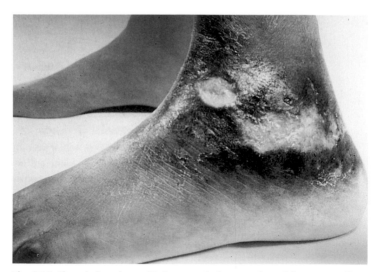

Fig. 3.11 Chronic leg ulcer with increased pigmentation of the surrounding skin in a woman with sickle-cell anaemia.

adults and progress to renal failure. Chronic renal failure is encountered especially after the age of 40 years and is caused by a combination of cortical and medullary infarction, glomerular sclerosis, tubular damage and infection. The prevalence of subfertility in males is increased. In females, pregnancy may be associated with a worsening of symptoms and there is an increased occurrence of peripartum fetal loss.

There is a high early mortality rate, the magnitude of which is dependent on the quality of health care and on living conditions. In a prospective survey in Jamaica, 13% of the children died in the first 2 years of life (Sergeant 1985). The principal causes of death were acute splenic sequestration of red cells and pneumococcal sepsis (meningitis, pneumonia, septicaemia), both of extremely rapid onset, but both amenable to treatment.

Diagnosis
Many patients with sickle-cell anaemia have at least a few sickled cells in their blood film (Plate 6) but others do not. The diagnosis is made by finding (a) a positive result with a screening test for HbS; (b) a single major band moving in the position of HbS on electrophoresis both at an alkaline and acid pH (see Fig. 3.6); and (c) the sickle-cell trait in both parents. The screening tests for HbS-containing red cells are based on the decreased solubility of deoxygenated HbS; they involve the detection of sickling after mixing with the reducing agent sodium metabisulphite (sickling test) or the development of turbidity after addition to a lysis buffer containing the reducing agent sodium dithionite (sickle solubility test). Heterozygotes for HbS also give a positive result with these screening tests but do not have sickled cells on their blood films, and show a mixture of HbA and S on electrophoresis.

Treatment
Principles of management of sickle-cell anaemia include:
1 immunization with pneumococcal vaccine and treatment with prophylactic penicillin V to minimize the risk from fulminant infections;
2 administration of folic acid daily to prevent secondary folate deficiency;
3 avoidance of factors precipitating painful crises such as dehydration, hypoxia, circulatory stasis and cooling of the skin;
4 active treatment for bacterial infections that may precipitate or have precipitated crises;
5 treatment of painful crises with oral or intravenous fluids and analgesics, including morphine when necessary;

6 early detection of pulmonary sickling (blood gas measurements and chest X-ray) and the administration of O_2 by mask in hypoxic patients, and

7 blood transfusion in certain circumstances.

Transfusion is indicated for visceral sequestration and aplastic crises. Exchange transfusions are useful in certain situations, particularly in severe pulmonary crises, in priapism, when there is evidence of neurological damage and when crises occur very frequently. In the latter situation, exchange transfusion should be followed by regular blood transfusion to keep the HbS level below 40%; patients who are regularly transfused for prolonged periods ($> 1–2$ years) must receive desferrioxamine to prevent iron overload. Regular transfusion may be required during pregnancy in patients with frequent crises or a poor obstetric history.

A number of children with sickle-cell anaemia have been cured by bone marrow transplantation. The transplantation-related mortality appears to be low and the major problem with this procedure is graft failure. Recently, prolonged therapy with hydroxyurea, which increases HbF production, has been shown to cause a significant reduction in the incidence of severe crises. Increased γ-chain synthesis has a beneficial effect because it leads to the formation of $\alpha_2\gamma\beta^S$ molecules which do not participate in polymer formation with $\alpha_2\beta^S_2$ on deoxygenation.

Haemoglobins E and C

Both HbE and C result from single amino acid substitutions in the β-chains.

Haemoglobin E is very common in South-East Asia and is found in about 50% of the population in some parts of Thailand. Heterozygotes have about 20–30% HbE, are asymptomatic, and are usually not anaemic. They have a low mean cell volume (MCV) because the single base substitution in the β-globin gene creates an alternative splicing site in the primary mRNA transcript and, consequently, there is reduced production of mature mRNA for β^E-chains and reduced β^E-chain synthesis. Their blood films may contain a few target cells. Homozygotes are characterized by mild anaemia, a low MCV and many circulating target cells.

HbC is confined to people of West African extraction, being present in 7% and 22% of the population in Nigeria and northern Ghana, respectively. Heterozygotes have 30–40% HbC, are asymptomatic and non-anaemic, having 6–40% target cells in their blood. Homozygotes have a mild anaemia, low or normal MCV, splenomegaly and many target cells (Fig. 3.12).

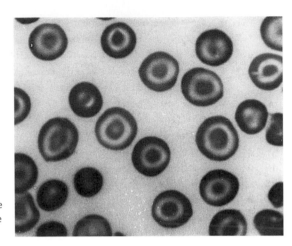

Fig. 3.12 Target cells in the blood film of a homozygote for HbC.

THALASSAEMIA

The thalassaemias are broadly divided into two main groups, the α-thalassaemias and the β-thalassaemias, depending on whether the defect lies in the synthesis of α- or β-globin chains, respectively (Weatherall & Clegg 1981).

α-Thalassaemias

The α-thalassaemias are seen with greatest frequency in South-East Asia (Thailand, Malay peninsula and Indonesia) and West Africa, the prevalence in these countries being 20–30%. They are also seen in southern Europe and the Middle East and sporadic cases have been reported in most racial groups. There are two closely linked α-globin genes on chromosome 16 and thus four α-globin genes per cell. In most patients with α-thalassaemia syndromes, the primary biochemical defect is a deletion of one, two, three or all four of the α-globin genes (Higgs & Weatherall 1993). However, dysfunctional rather than completely deleted genes are also occasionally found; these are caused by partial deletions or non-deletional defects (usually a single-base change). The manifestations of α-thalassaemia depend on the number of genes deleted in a particular individual. Deletion of one or two genes causes an asymptomatic condition with minor haematological changes; deletion of three and four genes causes HbH disease and Hb Bart's hydrops fetalis syndrome, respectively. There are two main varieties of abnormal chromosome (Fig. 3.13). In the first, one of the two genes on a chromosome may be deleted (α^+-thalassaemia determinant); in the second, both genes may be deleted (α^0-thalassaemia determinant). Both the α^0-thalassaemia and

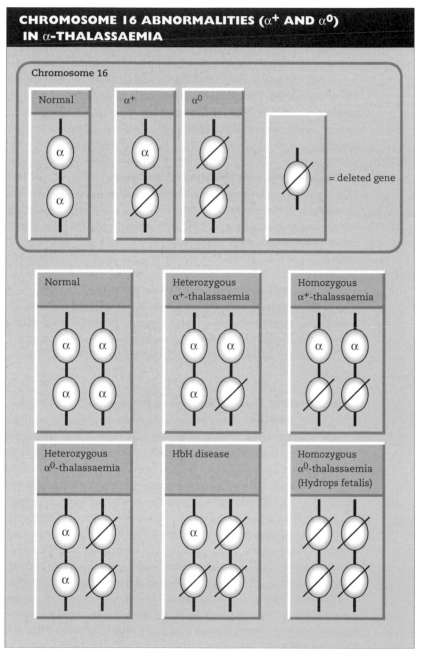

Fig. 3.13 Diagram to show how the two forms of abnormal chromosome 16 (α^+ and α^0) are arranged to give the different forms of α-thalassaemia. Homozygotes for α^0-thalassaemia suffer from Hb Bart's hydrops fetalis syndrome.

the α^+-thalassaemia determinants are found in South-East Asia and the Mediterranean region. The main type of α-thalassaemia determinant found in West Africa, the Middle East, India and the Pacific Islands is α^+; α^0 is very rare. In populations in which the α^0-thalassaemia determinant is rare, HbH disease is rare and Hb Bart's hydrops fetalis syndrome is not found. In Northern Thailand, where both the α^+ and α^0 determinants are particularly common, 0.4% of deliveries are stillbirths due to Hb Bart's hydrops fetalis syndrome and HbH disease is found in about 1% of the population.

α^+-Thalassaemia trait (deletion of one gene)
This condition is seen when the α^+-thalassaemia determinant is present on only one of the number 16 chromosomes (i.e. in heterozygotes for the α^+ determinant). Patients are asymptomatic but may be slightly anaemic. About 15% show slight reductions in MCV and mean cell Hb (MCH).

α^0-Thalassaemia trait (deletion of two genes)
This is seen in two circumstances, either in homozygotes for the α^+-thalassaemia determinant or in heterozygotes for the α^0-thalassaemia determinant. Similar haematological changes are seen in both situations. The Hb is either normal or slightly reduced and the MCV and MCH are usually reduced.

Haemoglobin H disease (deletion of three genes)
This chronic haemolytic anaemia results from the presence of both the α^+- and α^0-thalassaemia determinants. α-chains are produced at very low rates and there is a considerable excess of β-chains which combine to form tetramers (β_4). This tetramer is known as HbH. HbH is unstable and precipitates as the erythrocytes get older, forming rigid Heinz bodies (Plate 15) which are removed during passage of affected red cells through the spleen. The damage to the membrane brought about by this removal results in a shortened red-cell life-span. The clinical picture of HbH disease is very variable. Most patients are moderately affected with a condition similar to β-thalassaemia intermedia, some are more severely affected and others are only mildly affected and live almost normal lives. Splenomegaly is seen in most patients. The Hb concentration is usually between 7 and 11 g/dl but may be as low as 3–4 g/dl; the red cells are hypochromic and show variation in size and shape. Both the MCV and MCH are reduced.

Hb Bart's hydrops fetalis syndrome (deletion of four genes)
This occurs when there is homozygosity for the α^0-thalassaemia determinant. No α-chains can be formed and the predominant chain synthesized is the γ-chain, which forms tetramers (γ_4, Hb Bart's). There is persistence in the fetus of the embryonic Hb, Hb Portland ($\zeta_2\gamma_2$) (p. 1). Intrauterine death followed by a stillbirth usually occurs between 25 and 40 weeks of gestation, or the baby dies very shortly after birth.

β-Thalassaemias
The prevalence of β-thalassaemia trait in southern Europe, South-East Asia and Africa is about 10–30%, 5% and 1.5%, respectively. The trait is also frequently seen in the Middle East, India, Pakistan and southern China. It has been suggested that the high prevalence of the β-thalassaemia gene in these regions results from the gene bestowing a protective effect against *Plasmodium falciparum* on heterozygotes.

The β-thalassaemias result from more than 125 different genetic abnormalities affecting the β-gene or the upstream promoter regions flanking the β-gene or the β-locus control region (p. 3); the prevalence of particular abnormalities varies between different races (Higgs & Weatherall 1993). When the β-chain genes are affected, they are usually not completely deleted but often show single nucleotide substitutions or additions, or small deletions. Patients in whom the genetic abnormality causes an absence of β-chain production are described as having β^0-thalassaemia, and those in whom the abnormality causes a reduction in the rate of β-chain production are described as having β^+-thalassaemia. The β^0-type predominates in India and Pakistan, the β^+-type predominates in Sardinia and Cyprus; both types are found in Greece, the Middle East and Thailand.

Mutations in the coding region of the β-gene may disrupt the normal reading frame (frame-shifts) or introduce a premature termination codon (nonsense mutations). Mutations may also affect the initiator codon, regions involved in RNA processing, the polyadenylation site or the CAP site (p. 3). In some β-thalassaemia mutations, no mRNA is produced at all, in others there is a reduced production, and in some, structurally and/or functionally abnormal mRNA is transcribed and sometimes, translated into structurally abnormal (truncated) β-chains that do not form viable tetramers.

Heterozygous β-thalassaemia
Most affected subjects are asymptomatic. The Hb concentration is either normal (thalassaemia minima) or slightly reduced (thalassaemia minor), the red-cell count is high and the MCV is usually low. The Romanowsky-

stained blood film shows microcytosis, target cells and red cells with basophilic stippling (i.e. several fine or coarse bluish-black granules consisting of aggregated ribosomes). The HbA_2 level is raised to 3.5–7.0% and half the cases show slightly increased HbF levels, which are in the range 1–5%. Serum iron, serum transferrin and serum ferritin are normal in the absence of co-existing iron deficiency.

Homozygous β-thalassaemia

This condition causes one of two syndromes, one characterized by severe anaemia usually developing between the second and twelfth months of life (β-thalassaemia major), and the other by moderate anaemia presenting after the age of 1–2 years (β-thalassaemia intermedia).

The inability to produce β-chains leads to the presence of an excess of α-chains (globin chain imbalance) in early and late polychromatic erythroblasts. The excess α-chains precipitate within the cells and this leads to an impairment of various cellular functions and the phagocytosis and degradation of a proportion of the precipitate-containing erythroblasts by bone marrow macrophages (ineffective erythropoiesis) (Wickramasinghe 1976). There is also a considerably shortened survival of precipitate-containing red cells which enter the circulation so that the anaemia results from a combination of ineffective erythropoiesis and peripheral haemolysis. The response to the anaemia and ineffective erythropoiesis is an enormous erythroid hyperplasia which results in skeletal changes mainly affecting the skull, long bones and hands.

β-thalassaemia major (Cooley's anaemia)

This disease does not present at birth since production of fetal Hb, $\alpha_2\gamma_2$, is not affected. The infant becomes profoundly anaemic (Hb concentration 2.5–6.5 g/dl) and mildly jaundiced after the first few months of life, at the time when HbA should be replacing HbF. There is also failure to thrive, abdominal enlargement due to hepatosplenomegaly, and recurrent fever. If a transfusion programme is not instituted, growth is retarded, the abdomen becomes more enlarged, muscle development is poor and various skeletal deformities due to the gross expansion of erythropoietic tissue appear. The skeletal changes cause the typical 'thalassaemic' facies with frontal and parietal bossing, enlargement of the maxillary bones causing severe dental deformities and malocclusion of the teeth, and depression of the bridge of the nose. The long bones and bones of the hands show thinning of the cortex. Fractures of long bones are frequent and may be the presenting sign. X-ray of the skull shows enlargement of the diploic spaces and radiating striations in the subperiosteal bone ('hair-on-end' appearance) (Fig. 3.2).

The excessive red-cell destruction (due to deposits of α-chain in the red cells) causes considerable enlargement of the spleen, and this itself may aggravate the anaemia due to increased pooling of red cells in that organ, an expanded plasma volume and secondary hypersplenism with a further shortening of red-cell life-span. The hypersplenism also causes neutropenia and thrombocytopenia.

Iron absorption from the gut is excessive, and this, together with the regular blood transfusions (each unit of blood contains 200 mg iron) causes secondary iron overload which, in the absence of long term iron chelation therapy, usually leads to death between the ages of 10 and 20 years. Iron deposition causes cirrhosis of the liver, diabetes mellitus and myocardial damage leading to fatal arrhythmias or congestive cardiac failure. The iron deposition also causes endocrine dysfunction and leads to a failure to grow normally during puberty and a failure to develop secondary sexual characteristics.

Diagnosis of β-thalassaemia major
The peripheral blood contains microcytic hypochromic red cells which also vary greatly in size and shape, and target cells (Fig. 3.14). Electrophoresis of Hb shows only or mainly HbF. There is an absence or reduction of HbA, depending on whether the abnormal genes are of the β^0 or β^+ type. The serum iron concentration is high, the serum transferrin concentration is usually slightly low and the transferrin is often completely saturated with iron. The serum ferritin level is increased, roughly in proportion to the extent of iron overload.

Treatment of β-thalassaemia major
It is not possible to appreciably alter globin chain production at the present time. Therefore therapy centres on regular transfusions, about every 4–6 weeks, so that the Hb concentration is always maintained above 11 g/dl. With this treatment, children grow and mature normally and lead normal lives. If the spleen is considerably enlarged and there is clear evidence that it is also trapping the transfused red cells and increasing transfusion requirements, splenectomy is carried out. An important aspect of modern treatment is the reduction of tissue damage due to secondary iron overload by the daily administration of the iron-chelating agent, desferrioxamine. This agent is given subcutaneously overnight using a portable pump and has been shown to limit iron accumulation and prolong life.

Recently, some patients have been successfully treated with bone

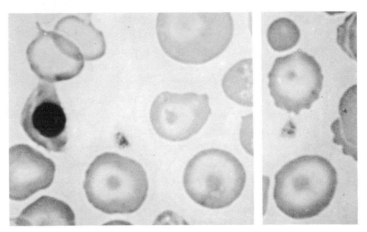

Fig. 3.14 Target cells, hypochromic red cells and an erythroblast from the peripheral blood film of a patient with homozygous β-thalassaemia.

marrow transplants from an HLA-matched sibling or parent. The procedure carries a mortality of 5–10% and in those who survive, the success rate is about 80%.

Antenatal diagnosis of β-thalassaemia major
It is possible to make an antenatal diagnosis of homozygous β-thalassaemia on blood obtained from an 18–20-week-old fetus. The reticulocytes are analysed for β-chain production and the diagnosis of homozygous β-thalassaemia is made when β-chain production is absent or markedly reduced. Parents often decide to abort homozygous fetuses. Antenatal diagnosis can be made much earlier during pregnancy from an analysis of chorionic villous DNA (at 9–12 weeks) or amniocyte DNA (at 13–16 weeks), either directly by using oligonucleotide probes complementary to specific mutations, or indirectly by linkage analysis with polymorphic restriction sites at the β-globin gene cluster.

β-thalassaemia intermedia
Most patients with this condition are reasonably well and require transfusions only during intercurrent infections. Clinical features include skeletal deformities (see p. 64), splenomegaly (which may become sufficiently marked to require splenectomy), formation of masses of extramedullary haemopoietic tissue which may cause pressure symptoms, recurrent leg ulcers, and haemosiderosis in adult life due to increased iron absorption. The clinical picture of β-thalassaemia intermedia is less severe than that of β-thalassaemia major because the extent of globin chain imbal-

Continued

ance (see p. 64) is smaller in the former that in the latter. The reduced chain imbalance may be a consequence of homozygosity for a 'mild' β^+-thalassaemia gene or of heterozygosity for both a β-thalassaemia gene and another genetic abnormality associated with mild chain imbalance such as Hb Lepore, HbE or $\delta\beta$-thalassaemia. Alternatively the extent of chain imbalance in homozygous β-thalassaemia may be reduced by co-inheritance of one or two α-thalassaemia genes or by increased γ-chain synthesis (e.g. caused by a mutation leading to hereditary persistence of HbF). As has been mentioned, the clinical picture of thalassaemia intermedia is also found in HbH disease (an α-thalassaemia syndrome).

Acquired haemolytic anaemias

Red cells may be destroyed either by immunological or by non-immunological mechanisms (Tabbara 1992).

IMMUNE HAEMOLYTIC ANAEMIAS

In these conditions, red cells react with antibody with or without complement activation and are consequently destroyed. IgG-coated red cells interact with the Fc receptors on macrophages and are then either completely or partially phagocytosed. When the phagocytosis is partial, the unphagocytosed part of the cell may detach from the macrophage and circulate as a spherocyte. Red cells which are also coated with the activated complement component C3 interact with C3 receptors on macrophages and are usually completely phagocytosed. In most instances where complement is activated, the cascade sequence only proceeds as far as C3 deposition on the cell surface. In a few instances, activation of complement is more intense and proceeds as far as deposition of the membrane attack complex (C5–C9) which results in intravascular haemolysis.

The immune haemolytic anaemias include haemolytic transfusion reactions (p. 244), haemolytic disease of the newborn (p. 252), autoimmune haemolytic anaemias and some drug-related haemolytic anaemias. In paroxysmal nocturnal haemoglobinuria, there is an acquired defect in the red-cell membrane which leads to complement-mediated haemolysis.

Autoimmune haemolytic anaemias

A classification of the autoimmune haemolytic anaemias is given in Table 3.4. The antibody found in these patients can be subdivided into two characteristic types, 'warm' antibody and 'cold' antibody (Dacie 1992). A 'warm' antibody reacts best with the red cell at 37°C and does not bring

AUTOIMMUNE HAEMOLYTIC ANAEMIAS

Caused by warm-reactive antibodies
Idiopathic
Secondary (chronic lymphocytic leukaemia, lymphoma, other malignant
  tumours, systemic lupus erythematosus (SLE))

Caused by cold-reactive antibodies
Cold haemagglutinin disease
  Idiopathic
  Secondary (*Mycoplasma pneumoniae* infection, infectious
    mononucleosis, lymphomas)

Paroxysmal cold haemoglobinuria
Idiopathic
Secondary (some viral infections, congential and tertiary syphilis)

Table 3.4 Classification of autoimmune haemolytic anaemias.

about agglutination. A 'cold' antibody reacts best only at a temperature below 32°C and usually agglutinates the red cells. The clinical picture associated with the two types is different.

Autoimmune haemolytic anaemia (AIHA) with warm-reactive antibodies

Patients are usually over the age of 50 years. In the idiopathic condition haemolysis dominates the clinical picture, and no evidence can be found of any other disease. In the secondary condition, the haemolysis is associated with a primary disease such as chronic lymphocytic leukaemia or systemic lupus erythematosus. In most patients the nature of the antigen on the red cell with which the autoantibody reacts cannot be determined, but in a few patients the antibody reacts with some of the antigens of the Rh system.

Symptoms are unrelated to ambient temperature. The clinical presentation is extremely variable. Some patients are very ill with an acute onset of severe anaemia; others have few or no symptoms and a mild chronic anaemia or even a compensated haemolytic state. Mild jaundice is common and splenomegaly is almost always found.

Haematological findings include anaemia, spherocytosis (Fig. 3.15), reticulocytosis, erythroblastaemia and neutrophil leucocytosis. IgG, complement components or both can usually be detected on the red cells using a direct antiglobulin test.

In most patients, the haemolysis can be reduced by treatment with prednisolone, which is initially given in high doses. If there is no response

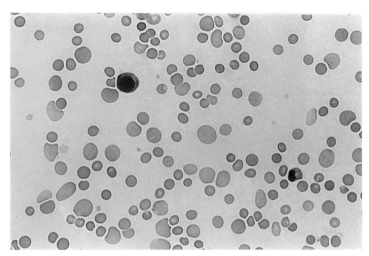

Fig. 3.15 Blood film from a patient with idiopathic autoimmune haemolytic anaemia (warm-reactive antibody). In addition to several microspherocytes, the photomicrograph shows two erythroblasts.

to steroids, or if the reduction in haemolysis is not maintained when the dose of steroids is decreased, splenectomy or immunosuppressive therapy with drugs such as azathioprine or cyclophosphamide should be tried and may be beneficial.

Cold haemagglutinin disease (CHAD)

Since cold antibody only reacts with red cells at a temperature below about 32°C, symptoms are worse during cold weather; skin temperature frequently falls well below 32°C when exposed to the cold. Exposure to cold provokes acrocyanosis (coldness, purplish discolouration and numbness of fingers, toes, ear lobes and the nose). This symptom is due to the formation of agglutinates of red cells in the vessels of the skin. Cold antibody attached to red cells also activates the complement system and leads to red-cell lysis and, consequently, to haemoglobinaemia and haemoglobinuria.

Blood films made at room temperature show large red-cell agglutinates (Fig. 3.16). The cold agglutinin in chronic idiopathic CHAD is usually a monoclonal IgM antibody usually with anti-I specificity. The anti-I titre at 4°C may be as high as 1:2000–1:500000 (normal, 1:10–40). (I and i are carbohydrate antigens expressed on red cells; adult red cells contain more I than i determinants.)

Rarely, patients with *Mycoplasma pneumonia* or infectious mononucleosis may develop acute self-limiting cold haemagglutinin disease due

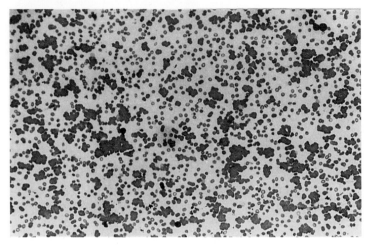

Fig. 3.16 Numerous red-cell agglutinates on a blood film from a patient with idiopathic cold haemagglutinin disease.

to the production of polyclonal IgM antibodies with anti-I or anti-i specificity, respectively.

Chronic idiopathic CHAD is treated by keeping the patient warm during the winter and, if necessary, by the use of chlorambucil or cyclophosphamide.

Paroxysmal cold haemoglobinuria

This rare disease is caused by an IgG antibody with anti-P specificity (P is a glycolipid red-cell antigen). This antibody is capable of binding complement and is called the Donath–Landsteiner antibody. Patients suffer from acute episodes of marked haemoglobinuria due to severe intravascular haemolysis when exposed to the cold. The diagnosis is based on serological studies demonstrating the presence of this particular antibody. A rapid screening test consists of incubating the patient's red cells and serum at 4°C and then warming the mixture to 37°C. Antibody and early complement components bind to red cells at 4°C but lysis occurs only on warming to 37°C (Donath–Landsteiner test).

Paroxysmal nocturnal haemoglobinuria (PNH)

This is an acquired disease in which an abnormal clone of haemopoietic cells derived from an abnormal haemopoietic stem cell gives rise to erythrocytes, leucocytes and platelets with defects in the cell membrane. At least nine membrane proteins, all of which are bound to the membrane by a glycosyl-phosphatidylinositol (GPI) anchor, are either missing or reduced because of a defect in the synthesis of the GPI anchor. At

Continued

least two of the membrane proteins affected (decay-accelerating factor or DAF and the membrane inhibitor of reactive lysis or MIRL) are concerned with the modulation of complement activation and, therefore, protection of the cells against inadvertent complement-mediated lysis. The affected cells are thus unusually sensitive to lysis by the terminal complement complex (C5–C9). The essential features of the disease are intravascular haemolysis, recurrent venous thrombosis and pancytopenia. The haemolysis is usually mild and chronic but may be severe and episodic with haemoglobulinuria, which is predominantly nocturnal. The PNH defect may occasionally develop during the course of aplastic anaemia. It may also precede marrow aplasia or develop after recovery from aplasia. Some cases of PNH terminate in acute leukaemia. The diagnosis is usually based on the susceptibility of PNH red cells to undergo lysis when incubated with acidified fresh autologous serum (acidified serum lysis test or Ham test).

NON-IMMUNE HAEMOLYTIC ANAEMIAS

Several of the causes of acquired non-immune haemolytic anaemia are summarized in Table 3.5. These include aortic valve prostheses (Plate 44), malaria (Fig. 3.17, Plate 46) and certain drugs.

Haemolytic anaemia due to drugs

Any drug which affects essential structural components or functional activities of a red cell is likely to cause a shortening of red-cell life-span. It is not surprizing, therefore, that a large number of drugs have been reported to cause haemolysis. When any haemolytic anaemia is encountered, it is necessary to enquire closely to determine whether there has been any exposure to drugs or chemicals (Worlledge et al. 1982; Murphy & Kelton 1991). Some drugs cause haemolysis by non-immune mechanisms and others by immune mechanisms.

The precise way in which many drugs act on the red cell is not known, but four categories of action can be recognized.

1 Certain chemicals, such as benzene, toluene and saponin, which are fat solvents, act on the red-cell membrane and disrupt its lipid components.

2 Certain drugs, such as primaquine, sulphonamides and phenacetin oxidize and denature Hb and other cell components in people with a deficiency of G6PD or some other red-cell enzymes (p. 47). However, if given in a large enough dose these drugs also affect normal red cells. When given in conventional doses, the two oxidant drugs dapsone and sulphasalazine cause haemolysis in most patients.

3 There are drugs which combine with components on the surface of the red cell and generate complexes which act as antigens. The resulting

NON-IMMUNE HAEMOLYSIS

MECHANICAL TRAUMA TO RED CELLS
Abnormalities in the heart and large blood vessels:
Aortic valve prostheses (Plate 44), severe aortic valve disease, extensive dissecting aneurysms of the aorta

Microangiopathic haemolytic anaemia:
Haemolytic uraemic syndrome, thrombotic thrombocytopenic purpura, metastatic malignancy, malignant hypertension, disseminated intravascular coagulation

March haemoglobinuria

BURNS

INFECTIONS
Clostridium perfringens (welchii), malaria (Fig. 3.17, Plate 46), bartonellosis

DRUGS*, CHEMICALS AND VENOMS
Oxidant drugs and chemicals, arsine, venoms of certain spiders and snakes

HYPERSPLENISM

* Some drugs cause haemolysis by immune mechanisms.

Table 3.5 Causes of acquired non-immune haemolytic anaemias.

antibody then reacts with the drug–cell surface complex and brings about red-cell destruction. Penicillin, when given in very large doses (more than 6 g/day), can occasionally cause a haemolytic anaemia in this way.

It was once considered that certain drugs become antigenic after combining with serum proteins. The antibodies produced were thought to form circulating antigen–antibody complexes which become adsorbed onto the red-cell surface. The adsorbed antigen–antibody complexes appeared to activate complement and cause lysis of the affected red cells (the 'innocent-bystander' mechanism). This mechanism of haemolysis was initially proposed for drugs such as stibophen and quinidine, but recent data indicate that such drugs attach with low affinity to the red-cell surface and that the drug-dependent antibodies have a specificity not only for the drug but also for red-cell membrane constituents.

4 Methyldopa and mefenamic or flufenamic acid trigger the development of an autoimmune haemolytic anaemia associated with warm-reactive autoantibodies, perhaps by an effect of the drug on suppressor T-lymphocytes.

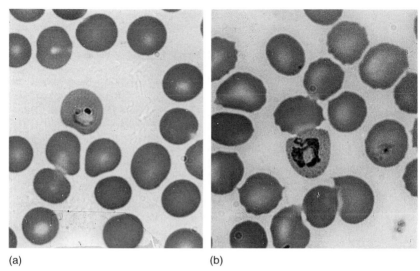

(a)   (b)

Fig. 3.17 Peripheral blood film from a patient with *Plasmodium vivax*
malaria showing two parasitized red cells each containing a single parasite.
(a) Ring form (early trophozoite) within a slightly enlarged red cell. (b)
Amoeboid late trophozoite; the parasitized cell is enlarged and stippled.
The ring forms of *Plasmodium falciparum* are smaller and more delicate than
those of *Plasmodium vivax* and do not cause enlargement of the parasitized
red cells (Plate 46). In falciparum malaria especially, more than one
parasite may be found within a single red cell.

Hypersplenism

The term 'hypersplenism' is used to describe the reduction in the life-
span of red cells, granulocytes and platelets that may be found in patients
with splenomegaly due to any cause. The cytopenias found in patients
with enlarged spleens are also partly caused by increased pooling of
blood cells within the spleen and an increased plasma volume; the
magnitude of both these effects is proportioned to spleen size. In some
haematological diseases in which anaemia is caused by a congenital or
acquired defect of the red cell or impaired red-cell formation, increasing
splenomegaly may result in increasing anaemia by the mechanisms mentioned above.

References

Dacie J. (1992) *The Haemolytic Anaemias*, 3rd edn, Vol 3: The Auto-Immune Haemolytic
Anaemias. Churchill Livingstone, Edinburgh.
Higgs D.R., Weatherall D.J. (eds.) (1993) *The Haemoglobinopathies*. Baillières Clinical
Haematology, International Practice and Research, Vol 6/No 1. Ballière Tindall,
London.

Lehmann H., Huntsman R.G. (1974) *Man's Haemoglobins*. North Holland Publishing Company, Amsterdam.

Mackinney A.A. (1965) Hereditary spherocytosis. *Arch. Intern. Med.* **116**, 257–265.

Mentzer W.C. (ed.) (1981) Enzymopathies. *Clinics in Haematology*, Vol 10.1. W.B. Saunders, Philadelphia.

Mollison P.L., Engelfriet C.P., Contreras M. (1987) *Blood Transfusion in Clinical Medicine*, 8th edn. Blackwell Scientific Publications, Oxford.

Murphy W.G., Kelton J.G. (1991) Immune haemolytic anaemia and thrombocytopenia: drugs and autoantibodies. *Biochem. Soc. Trans.* **19**, 183–186.

Palek J., Jarolim P. (1993) Clinical expression and laboratory detection of red cell membrane protein mutations. *Semin. Hematol.* **30**, 249–283.

Sergeant G.R. (1985) *Sickle-Cell Disease*. Oxford University Press, Oxford.

Tabbara I.A. (1992) Hemolytic anemias. Diagnosis and management. *Med. Clin. North. Am.* **76**, 649–668.

Vulliamy T., Mason P., Luzzatto L. (1992) The molecular basis of glucose-6-phospate dehydrogenase deficiency. *Trends Genet.* **8**, 138–143.

Weatherall D.J., Clegg J.B. (1981) *The Thalassaemia Syndromes*, 3rd edn. Blackwell Scientific Publications, Oxford.

Wickramasinghe S.N. (1976) The morphology and kinetics of erythropoiesis in homozygous β-thalassaemia. In: Porter R., Fitzsimons D.W. (eds.) *Congenital Disorders of Erythropoiesis*, Ciba Foundation Symposium 37 (new proceedings of series), pp. 221–243. Elsevier, Amsterdam.

Worlledge S., Hughes-Jones N.C., Bain B. (1982) Immune haemolytic anaemias. In: Hardisty R.M., Weatherall D.J. (eds.) *Blood and its Disorders*, p. 479. Blackwell Scientific Publications, Oxford.

Reviews

Allgood J.W., Chaplin H. (1967) Idiopathic acquired autoimmune hemolytic anemia. A review of forty-seven cases treated from 1955 through 1965. *Am. J. Med.* **43**, 254–273.

Dacie J. (1985) The Haemolytic Anaemias, 3rd edn, Vol 1: *The Hereditary Anaemias*, Part 1. Churchill Livingstone, Edinburgh.

Dacie J. (1988) The Haemolytic Anaemias, 3rd edn, Vol 2: *The Hereditary Anaemias*, Part 2. Churchill Livingstone, Edinburgh.

Kazazian H.H., Jr., Dowling C.E., Waber P.G., Huang S., Lo W.H.Y. (1986) The spectrum of β-thalassaemia genes in China and Southeast Asia. *Blood* **68**, 964–966.

Lee G.R., Bithell T.C., Foerster J., Athens J.W., Lukens J.N. (1993) *Wintrobe's Clinical Hematology*, 9th edn, Vols 1 & 2. Lea & Febiger, Philadelphia.

Lehmann H., Kynoch P.A.M. (1976) *Human Haemoglobin Variants and their Characteristics*. North Holland Publishing Company, Amsterdam.

Mentzer W.C. (ed.) (1981) Enzymopathies. *Clinics in Haematology*, Vol 10.1. W.B. Saunders, Philadelphia.

Nagel R.L. (ed.) (1991) *Hemoglobinopathies*. Hematology/Oncology Clinics of North America, Vol 5/No 3. W.B. Saunders, Philadelphia.

Van dem Borne A.E.G.Kr. (ed.) (1991) Molecular immunohaematology. *Clin. Haematol.* **4**, 793–1014.

CHAPTER 4

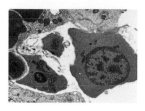

Iron Metabolism, Iron-Deficiency Anaemia and other Hypochromic Microcytic Anaemias

Objectives in learning

1 To know about the dietary sources, mechanism of absorption, site of storage and method of plasma transportation of iron and the mechanism and extent of iron loss in men and women.

2 To know the causes of iron deficiency at all ages and in both sexes.

3 To know the stages of iron deficiency and progression from iron depletion to iron-deficiency anaemia.

4 To know the mode of presentation of iron-deficiency anaemia.

5 To know the changes in the morphology of the red cells, in the red-cell indices, in the plasma iron levels and in the bone marrow associated with iron deficiency.

6 To know how to differentiate between the anaemia due to chronic disorders and that due to iron deficiency.

7 To know the principles of treatment of iron deficiency, both by the oral and parenteral routes.

8 To know the causes of hypochromic microcytic red cells other than iron deficiency.

9 To understand the causes and consequences of iron overload.

Iron-deficiency anaemia is the most common type of anaemia throughout the world affecting about 25% of the world population. Its prevalence in poor countries is considerably higher than in rich countries. Iron-deficiency anaemia is an important world health problem for three main reasons (Dallman 1989; Parks & Wharton 1989). Firstly, anaemia in pregnancy (due mainly to iron deficiency) is associated with an increased risk of low birth weight, prematurity and perinatal mortality. Secondly, there is good evidence that infants and children with iron-deficiency anaemia have impaired psychomotor development and cognitive performance; iron replacement has both immediate and long-term beneficial effects. Thirdly, iron deficient people have a decreased work capacity.

Metabolism of iron

DISTRIBUTION OF IRON IN THE BODY

Essential iron-containing compounds are found in the plasma and in all cells. Since ionized iron is toxic, virtually all of the iron is present within the haem moiety of a haemoprotein (e.g. haemoglobin (Hb), myoglobin (Mb) and cytochrome) or directly bound to a protein (e.g. transferrin, ferritin and haemosiderin). The total body iron content of a healthy adult varies between 2 and 5 g. About two-thirds of this iron is found in the Hb of red cells: since 1 ml of red cells contains approximately 1 mg of iron, an adult has about 2 g of iron in the red-cell mass. About 0.15 g of iron is present in the Mb of muscle cells and in the respiratory enzymes of all cells. Most of the remainder of the iron is stored in the macrophages of the spleen and bone marrow and in both the Kupffer and parenchymal cells of the liver. The stores of iron vary from 0 to 1 g or more. Storage iron exists in the two forms, ferritin and haemosiderin. Ferritin is water-soluble and is composed of a protein shell which encloses an iron core containing up to 4500 atoms of iron. Haemosiderin is insoluble and is composed of aggregates of ferritin molecules which have partly lost their protein shell. Haemosiderin appears as golden-brown granules in unstained preparations or as blue granules inside macrophages when stained by Perls' acid ferrocyanide method (Prussian Blue reaction). As ferritin is water soluble, it is leached out during the preparation of histological sections and is not detectable by the Prussian Blue reaction.

DYNAMIC STATE OF BODY IRON

Iron is continuously circulating through the plasma bound to the protein, transferrin. The major part of this circulating iron is derived from the daily destruction of approximately 20 ml of red cells, which liberate 20 mg of iron (Fig. 4.1). There is also a further 5 mg of iron carried through the plasma daily. This iron is derived from the iron stores and from absorption in the gastrointestinal tract. Plasma iron is rapidly removed, mainly by erythropoietic tissue in the bone marrow, but part goes to other dividing cells and to the iron stores. The half-time for passage of iron through the circulation depends on the plasma iron concentration and varies between 50 and 110 minutes.

IRON ABSORPTION

Iron is present in both vegetables and meat and although the concentration is higher in the latter, the iron content of the diet of most

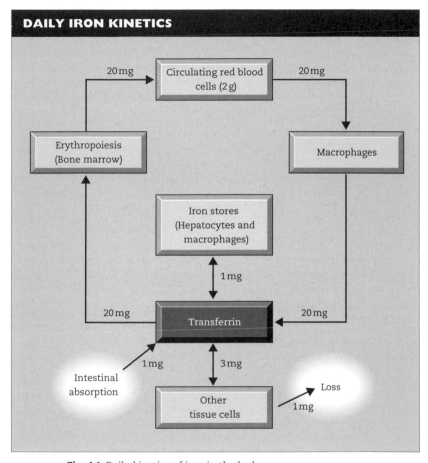

DAILY IRON KINETICS

Fig. 4.1 Daily kinetics of iron in the body.

vegetarians is adequate and the incidence of iron-deficiency anaemia no greater than in omnivores. However, macrobiotic or vegan diets with a high phytate and fibre content do result in a greater incidence of iron deficiency. An average omnivorous diet contains approximately 10–20 mg of iron per day, mostly in ferric–protein complexes and haem–protein complexes but also in inorganic form.

Adults who have normal iron stores absorb approximately 5–10% of their total intake, i.e. they absorb 0.5–2 mg/day. Iron is absorbed in the upper half of the small intestine. The haem molecule is absorbed best; it is taken up by intestinal epithelial cells within which the iron is split from the porphyrin ring. Non-haem iron is less well absorbed as it can be readily bound and made non-absorbable by ligands such as phytate and phosphate that are found in food; its absorption is promoted by gastric HCl. Ferric iron must be reduced to the ferrous form before absorption; hence oral iron is given therapeutically as the ferrous salt. Ascorbic acid promotes the absorption of non-haem iron, partly because it is a reducing agent and partly because it forms a molecular complex with it, which is readily absorbed.

The prevalence of gastric atrophy and of achlorhydria is higher in patients with iron-deficiency anaemia than in healthy people. It is probable that the gastric atrophy is the primary event and that the consequent achlorhydria is an aetiological factor in the development of iron deficiency. In most instances, the gastric mucosa does not return to normal after cure of the iron deficiency.

Absorption of iron does not remain constant at 5–10% of total intake but is inversely related to the size of iron stores and directly related to the rate of erythropoiesis. When iron intake is in excess of that required for growth and to replenish the daily loss of iron from the body, iron is stored in the liver, spleen and bone marrow. As iron stores increase, the rate of accumulation in the stores decreases, mainly due to a slowing in the rate of absorption. Eventually an equilibrium is reached when iron stores remain constant. On the other hand, when iron stores decrease, the absorptive mechanism is stimulated and the percentage of iron absorbed is increased so that, in iron deficiency, absorption may rise to over 50% of the total intake.

Iron that enters from the gut contents into the epithelial cells is either passed on to the plasma transferrin or remains within the cells and combines with apoferritin to form ferritin. The transfer of iron from the epithelial cells into the plasma is controlled by an unidentified mechanism which responds to iron requirements, the rate being rapid when stores are reduced or the rate of erythropoiesis is increased. Iron not transferred to the plasma remains in the epithelial cells until desquamation takes place and the iron is then excreted in the faeces.

IRON LOSS

There is no specific excretory mechanism for iron. Nevertheless, there is an inevitable daily loss of iron as a result of the continuous exfoliation of gut and skin epithelial cells, all of which have iron-containing enzymes. In adults, this loss is approximately 1 mg/day. The extra loss in women due to menstruation and pregnancy is discussed later (p. 82)

Iron-depletion and iron-deficiency anaemia

As body iron stores are depleted, three phases can be recognized. The first stage is depletion of iron stores without diminished iron supply to tissues and without anaemia. Further depletion of body iron results in a reduced iron supply to tissues. Eventually this leads to a fall in Hb concentration and the picture of iron-deficiency anaemia. Iron depletion without anaemia is far more common than iron-deficiency anaemia. Thus in one study (Hallberg et al. 1993a), only 6% of iron depleted women had Hb levels below 12 g/dl, and in another study, about a quarter of those with iron depletion were also anaemic.

PREVALENCE OF IRON DEFICIENCY

Iron-deficiency anaemia is the most common haematological abnormality and probably the commonest non-infectious disorder throughout the world. Although more frequently found among the poor due to in-adequate dietary intake, it is also prevalent among the affluent. Iron-deficiency anaemia appears most frequently during three periods of life; namely, in infants of both sexes, in women during the child-bearing period, and in the elderly. The following is a brief summary of recent reports of its prevalence in several parts of the world.

Prevalence in infancy

Two reports demonstrate the high frequency of iron deficiency in infancy. A study on 0.5–3-year-old infants in a socially deprived urban area in New Zealand found that 23% had iron-deficiency anaemia (Hb concentration < 11.0 g/dl) (Crampton et al. 1994), and a study on healthy Asian children in the UK found that 17% were anaemic (Duggan et al. 1991). The importance of diagnosing and treating iron-deficiency anaemia in infants is shown by the recent findings that anaemic infants are not as successful in tests of mental and motor development as their normal counterparts. Treatment with iron has been found to reverse these changes (Sheard 1994).

Prevalence in primary school children

By the age of 5–6 years, iron-deficiency anaemia is relatively uncommon, being found in only 1 per 378 children in a primary school in the UK. However, 2% were iron depleted (serum ferritin < 8 μg/l) (Hammond et al. 1994).

Prevalence in adolescents

By the age of 15–16 years iron depletion again becomes common. Studies in Sweden, Australia and Canada have all provided similar findings; namely about 40% of girls and 15% of boys are iron depleted (serum ferritin < 16 μg/l) (Hallberg et al. 1993b).

Prevalence in women of child-bearing age

Loss of iron to the fetus and through lactation, in addition to menstruation, results in a relatively high incidence of iron depletion and deficiency in this group of people. In 1993, a Danish survey of premenopausal women found 12% to be depleted (serum ferritin < 20 μg/l) and 3% to be anaemic (Hb < 12 g/dl) (Milman et al. 1993).

Prevalence in males, 30–60 years old

As there is no physiological iron loss in this group other than desquamation from skin and gut, iron deficiency is uncommon. A Danish survey (Milman & Kirchhoff 1991) found that only 5% were depleted and only about 1 per 700 were anaemic.

Prevalence in the elderly

Many studies on the elderly in Europe have shown that the prevalence of iron-deficiency anaemia is relatively high, varying between 2 and 10% in both sexes (Joosten et al. 1993).

CAUSES OF IRON DEFICIENCY

Iron stores become depleted when the rate of absorption of iron is insufficient to replace iron lost from the body. Inadequate absorption may be due to a low iron content of the diet or to impairment of intestinal absorptive mechanisms. On the other hand, loss of iron through haemorrhage may occur at a greater rate than it can be replaced. The causes of iron deficiency are summarized in Table 4.1.

Causes of iron deficiency related to the gastrointestinal tract

A review of 378 in-patients with an iron-deficiency anaemia (Beveridge et al. 1965) revealed that gastrointestinal bleeding accounted for 40% of the cases, with a poor diet, gastrectomy and steatorrhoea each accounting for a further 10–20%. Bleeding from various lesions in the upper gastrointestinal tract is about three times as common as from lesions in the colon (Rockey & Cello 1993).

Gastrectomy carried out by the Polya method (common before 1960) is frequently followed by iron deficiency. In one study, 40% of patients were iron deficient (transferrin saturation < 16%) 9–14 years

CAUSES OF IRON DEFICIENCY

Reduced iron stores at birth due to prematurity

Inadequate intake (prolonged breast or bottle feeding without iron supplementation, vegetarian diets, poverty)

Increased requirement (pregnancy and lactation)

Chronic haemorrhage
  Uterine (menorrhagia, metrorrhagia)
  Gastrointestinal (e.g. hiatus hernia, oesophageal varices, peptic
    ulceration, Meckel's diverticulum, colonic diverticulosis, ulcerative
    colitis, carcinoma of the stomach, colon or rectum, haemorrhoids,
    hereditary telangiectasia – see p. 208, hookworm infestation*)
  Other (e.g. self-inflicted, recurrent haematuria)

Malabsorption (coeliac disease, partial gastrectomy)

Chronic intravascular haemolysis leading to haemoglobinuria and
haemosiderinuria (rare)

* This is a very common cause of iron deficiency in tropical countries.

Table 4.1

after a partial gastrectomy, and by the third decade post-gastrectomy 70–90% were iron deficient (Tovey et al. 1990). Iron deficiency in these patients is due to inadequate absorption, probably due to an abnormally rapid rate of passage of food through the upper part of the small intestine. In addition, bleeding from the mucosal remnant of the stomach has also been observed, sometimes at a rate of over 150 ml of blood per month (Holt et al. 1970). The malabsorption syndrome (e.g. in coeliac disease) also frequently causes iron deficiency and iron-deficiency anaemia.

Causes of iron deficiency in infancy

There are two factors which predispose to iron deficiency in infancy; namely, inadequate iron stores at birth, and inadequate amounts of iron in the diet. The amount of iron derived from the mother is dependent on her iron status. A child born to an iron deficient mother is about six times as likely to develop iron-deficiency anaemia compared to a mother with adequate iron stores (Colomer et al. 1990). As about half the iron stores are deposited in the last month of fetal life, premature babies may deplete their iron stores before starting on iron-rich solid food. The growing child needs to absorb 0.5–1.0 mg of iron each day during the first year (Burman 1982); this cannot be supplied by either human or cow's milk, since both sources have low concentrations of iron and five to nine pints would be required to provide sufficient iron for the child's daily needs.

Infants that are not breast fed should therefore be given an iron supplemented milk formula. Furthermore, when solids are introduced, all infants should be given iron-fortified foods (e.g. infant cereal). The value of iron supplementation is shown by a survey made in the UK (Mills 1990) of children aged 8–24 months, where it was found that 22% had iron-deficiency anaemia. All these anaemic cases were associated with prolonged feeding with breast or cow's milk. In contrast, no cases of anaemia were found in those who had been fed formula milk.

Causes of iron deficiency in women of child-bearing age
The prevalence of iron deficiency is high in women because of excessive loss of iron through menstruation and child bearing.

Iron loss through menstruation
The measurement of blood loss during menstruation shows that the rate of loss in many women is sufficient to reduce the iron stores rapidly. It has been observed (Hallberg et al. 1966) that most women losing more than 60 ml of blood with each period were either iron depleted or had iron-deficiency anaemia. A study of the monthly menstrual blood loss in normal women showed a range from less than 10 ml to 180 ml (Fig. 4.2) (Jacobs et al. 1965). The diagram also indicates the approximate iron requirements (assuming absorption of 10% of the dietary iron) and it can be seen that women losing 60 ml of blood require about 20 mg of iron in their daily diet, which is about the maximum contained in a normal diet.

Causes of iron deficiency in pregnancy
Hb concentration falls in pregnancy and normal lower limits have been variously reported to be between 10 and 12 g/dl; the World Health Organization (WHO) has recommended that a lower normal limit of 11 g/dl should be taken for practical purposes. The main reason for this fall is an increase in plasma volume; red-cell mass increases by 200–500 ml but there is an even greater increase in plasma volume resulting in haemodilution. This increase in red-cell mass requires an extra 200–500 mg of iron, but this is offset by the fact that there is a reduction in iron loss by approximately the same amount due to amenorrhoea.

The total amount of iron required by the mother during each pregnancy is high, being of the order of 500–700 mg. The fetus requires approximately 250 mg; the rest is lost in the placenta and through

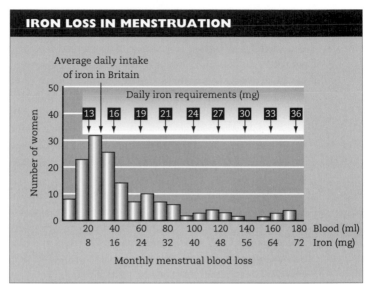

Fig. 4.2 Menstrual blood loss in 151 normal women. The daily iron
requirements are calculated on the basis that 10% of the iron in the diet
is absorbed. (After Jacobs et al. 1965.)

haemorrhage; the average blood loss during parturition is of the order of
300 ml (Newton et al. 1961). Thus, pregnant women require to absorb
each day about 2–3 mg more than when not pregnant. This is more than
can be absorbed from a normal unsupplemented diet, and unless the
mother starts pregnancy with more than about 200 mg of storage iron,
iron depletion will almost certainly occur.

A survey of pregnant women in Canada revealed that about 25% of
the mothers were iron depleted (serum ferritin < 15 μg/l) at the time of
delivery. In another study, 90% of Danish women had serum ferritin
values less than 20 μg/l at term and 17% had iron-deficiency anaemia
(Godel et al. 1992). Iron supplementation (65 mg iron/day) from the
second trimester prevented iron-deficiency anaemia (Milman et al. 1994).

CLINICAL PRESENTATION

Symptoms

Iron-deficiency anaemia develops slowly, thereby permitting various
adaptive mechanisms to operate and compensate for the effects of the
developing anaemia (p. 25). Consequently, symptoms are usually only
seen when Hb falls below about 8 g/dl. Various symptoms referable to the

cardiovascular and nervous system such as malaise, fatigue, faintness, lack of concentration, dizziness, irritability, headache, palpitations, breathlessness, swelling of ankles and pain in the chest, are reported by some patients with Hb values between 8 and 12 g/dl. However, these symptoms can clearly be caused by a great variety of other diseases and are common in neurosis. It has been shown (Berry & Nash 1954) that this type of symptom is common in people without anaemia and, conversely, many people with mild anaemia (Hb values of 10–12 g/dl) do not have symptoms.

Peculiar dietary cravings (pica), e.g. for soil or ice, may be found in some cases of iron-deficiency anaemia.

The combination of post-cricoid dysphagia, associated in some cases with a web or stricture, atrophic glossitis and iron-deficiency anaemia is known as the Paterson–Kelly or Plummer–Vinson syndrome. The dysphagia, web and anaemia disappear after iron therapy. It has been suggested that the dysphagia could be due to a deficiency of iron-containing compounds in the epithelial cells lining the pharyngo-oesophageal junction or in muscle fibres involved in swallowing.

Signs

The signs of anaemia are discussed on p. 26. In addition to these, the following signs resulting from a deficiency of iron in epithelial tissues may be found: redness of the tongue and loss of papillae (glossitis); abnormal nails, either spoon-shaped (koilonychia) or flat; and angular stomatitis. For unknown reasons, these signs of epithelial iron deficiency are less frequently seen today than in the past. The tip of the spleen is palpable in about 10% of cases.

Haematological changes

Patients with mild anaemia may initially have a normal mean cell volume (MCV), mean corpuscular Hb (MCH) and mean corpuscular Hb concentration (MCHC) with anisocytosis of red cells. Soon the red cells become microcytic, as shown by a fall in the MCV, and this is accompanied by a similar fall in the MCH. The concentration of Hb in each cell (MCHC) is thus unchanged initially. It is only at a later stage that the MCHC is reduced (when calculated from a microhaematocrit or measured on a Technicon HI series automated counter, p. 262). The MCHC is invariably reduced only when the Hb concentration falls below 7 g/dl in women and 9 g/dl in men (Beutler 1959).

Examination of a peripheral blood film usually shows red cells with hypochromia (p. 29), a reduced diameter (microcytosis) and increased variation in size (anisocytosis) and shape (poikilocytosis) (Fig. 4.3). Some

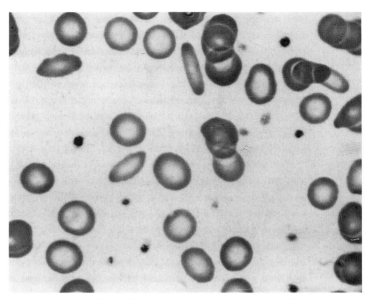

Fig. 4.3 Peripheral blood film from a patient with untreated iron deficiency anaemia. Hypochromic microcytes and elongated ('pencil-shaped') poikilocytes are present.

poikilocytes are elongated or pencil-shaped. Target cells may also be present.

A marrow smear stained by Perls' acid ferrocyanide method shows an absence of stainable iron in the macrophages within the bone marrow fragments (Plates 17 and 18). Erythropoiesis is normoblastic.

Assessment of iron stores

Serum iron concentration
The determination of serum iron concentration has been of considerable importance in establishing whether iron stores are depleted, but it suffers from three disadvantages: firstly, that there is a wide diurnal variation in the concentration (being lowest in the latter part of the day); secondly, concentrations are considerably lower during menstruation; and thirdly, the concentration is difficult to measure accurately. However, when the Hb concentration falls below 9 g/dl, the diurnal variation is less and the serum-iron concentration is usually consistently below 10 µmol/l.

Serum ferritin levels
The immunochemical measurement of the serum concentration of the

iron storage protein, ferritin, is now the method of choice for the diagnosis of iron deficiency. Ferritin is present in very small amounts in the serum and it has been found that its concentration roughly correlates with the amount of tissue storage iron, when the serum ferritin is below about 4000 µg/l. Within this range, a serum level of 100 µg/l represents about 1g of storage iron. However, there is no single value for ferritin concentration which clearly separates subjects with iron stores from subjects without, and there is a considerable overlap in ferritin levels between these two groups (Hallberg et al. 1993a) (Fig. 4.4). In the study illustrated in Fig. 4.4, all women with ferritin levels below 14 µg/l were iron deficient; on the other hand, 25% of the iron-deficient women had ferritin levels above this value. The higher level in these people is probably the result of biological variation, but in a small number of people results from the co-existence of acute and chronic infections or of malignancies which raise serum ferritin levels above that expected from the amount of storage iron. This increase in serum ferritin results from an increase in synthesis mediated by macrophage-derived inflammatory cytokines and nitric oxide.

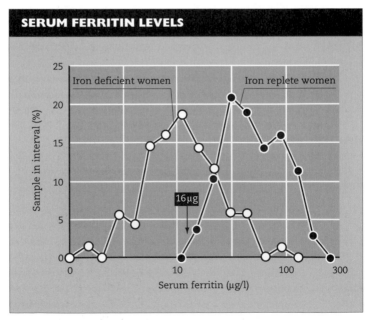

Fig. 4.4 Distribution of the serum ferritin concentration in 105 women with stainable iron in the bone marrow(●), and in 69 women with no stainable iron (○). (From Hallberg et al. 1993a.)

Transferrin concentration and extent of transferrin saturation

The concentration of the iron transport protein, transferrin, is frequently increased in iron deficiency. The transferrin concentration is now readily measured immunochemically. In the past it was measured indirectly by determining the maximum amount of iron that can be bound in serum, that is, the total iron binding capacity (TIBC). In iron-deficiency anaemia, the serum transferrin concentration is invariably raised when the Hb concentration falls below 9 g/dl, and is often raised when the Hb is in the range of 9–11 g/dl. Thus, a raised transferrin concentration is a useful diagnostic criterion, although the finding of raised levels in those taking oral contraceptives reduces its value considerably. The transferrin concentration is frequently reduced below normal in patients with infections, neoplasms and rheumatoid arthritis and thus helps to distinguish anaemia in these diseases from that due to iron deficiency.

An additional useful index is the extent of *transferrin saturation*, that is, the amount of iron bound to transferrin expressed as a percentage of the TIBC. Values of 16% or lower are usually found when there is an impaired supply of iron to the tissues as is the case in some individuals with lack of iron stores and in patients with iron-deficiency anaemia. Low values may also be found in the anaemia of chronic disorders.

Transferrin receptor

The recent introduction of the estimation of transferrin receptors in the serum by immunoassay has proved to be a very valuable method of distinguishing iron deficiency from the anaemia of chronic diseases (see p. 90). The transferrin receptor is present on all cells and iron gains entry by endocytosis following binding of the transferrin–iron complex to the receptor. A deficiency of iron results in an increase in the number of receptors on the red-cell surface. Small amounts of receptor are present in the plasma and the concentration reflects cellular receptor content. Transferrin receptor concentration rises two to three fold in iron deficiency; levels are not affected by conditions which give rise to the anaemia of chronic disease, nor are they affected by pregnancy (Cook *et al.* 1993).

DIAGNOSIS OF IRON DEPLETION WITHOUT ANAEMIA

When iron stores become depleted, a stage is reached when a stained marrow smear will show absent or virtually absent iron stores. At this time the serum ferritin concentration is usually less than 20 µg/ml. There may be some increase in serum transferrin but the serum iron concen-

IRON STATUS

| | Normal iron stores | Depleted iron stores | | |
		Without reduction of iron supply to tissues	Reduced iron supply to tissues, no anaemia	Iron-deficiency anaemia
Serum ferritin (μg/l)	20–300	usually <20	<20	<20
Transferrin (g/l)	1.7–3.4	sometimes >3.4	>3.4	>3.4
Serum iron (μmol/l)	10–30	Normal	<10	<10
Transferrin saturation (%)	>16	>16	<16	<16
Hb concentration	Normal	Normal	Within normal range	Below normal range

Table 4.2 Measurements of iron status in people with normal iron stores, individuals with iron depletion without anaemia and in iron-deficiency anaemia.

tration and the supply of iron to the tissues are within normal limits. With further depletion of body iron, there is a diminished iron supply to tissues and at this stage there is a reduction in both serum iron and transferrin saturation. Eventually, this leads to a reduction in iron compounds, particularly Hb concentration (Table 4.2).

Although the Hb concentration of a patient with depleted iron stores may be within the normal range, the value may be below the normal value for that person when iron stores are adequate.

TREATMENT OF IRON-DEFICIENCY ANAEMIA

Treatment should start with the oral administration of 200 mg anhydrous ferrous sulphate (containing 60 mg of elemental iron) three times daily. The minimal response in iron-deficient patients is a rise in Hb concentration of 2 g/dl in 3 weeks and most have rises in excess of this. The Hb concentration of the patient should therefore be measured again 3 weeks later to determine whether there has been an adequate response. If the patient has not responded the following points should be considered.

1 That the patient has not taken the tablets. One of the common reasons for not taking iron tablets is that the patient claims that they cause gastrointestinal symptoms, such as pain, diarrhoea or constipation. Those patients who cannot tolerate ferrous sulphate should be given another absorbable iron compound, e.g. ferrous gluconate, etc.

2 That the patient has the malabsorption syndrome.

3 If the iron deficiency was due to haemorrhage, this may still be operative, e.g. continued bleeding from the gut.

4 That vitamin B_{12} or folate deficiency is also present.

5 That the initial diagnosis was incorrect, e.g. the patient may have thalassaemia trait or the anaemia of chronic disorders rather than iron-deficiency anaemia.

The purpose of treatment with iron is not only to restore the Hb concentration to normal but also to replenish iron stores. The former is easy but the latter is difficult. The patient should therefore be persuaded to continue taking iron for 4–6 months after the Hb level becomes normal.

Patients with the malabsorption syndrome and those who cannot tolerate any form of iron orally, should receive iron parenterally. Either iron dextran (Imferon) or iron sorbitol (Jectofer) may be given daily by deep intramuscular injection, in a 10-day course. Frequently, the total amount of iron dextran required is given in a single intravenous infusion over 8–10 hours. Since life-threatening anaphylaxis may occur, the patient should receive a test dose prior to the infusion.

Although iron stores are usually absent in pregnancy, there is controversy as to whether all pregnant women should be treated with iron irrespective of their Hb concentration or only when the Hb falls below an arbitrary value (such as 11 g/dl, p. 82). The argument against treating all pregnant women with iron is that when this is done, haematological investigations are often omitted, so that other causes of anaemia (such as folate deficiency) are missed. Moreover, a considerable proportion of patients do not take the prescribed tablets, nor is the obstetrician informed of this. Some are of the opinion that it is safest to estimate the Hb concentration frequently and prescribe iron when required.

Other hypochromic microcytic anaemias

Hypochromic microcytic red cells are formed when there is a substantial impairment of the synthesis of the haem moiety or of the α- or β-globin chains of the Hb molecule. Iron deficiency is the most common cause of these changes; some of the other causes are listed in Table 4.3. Table 4.4 shows the way in which the three most common causes of hypochromia and microcytosis can be distinguished from each other on the basis of the

CAUSES OF HYPOCHROMIC MICROCYTIC RED CELLS

Iron deficiency

Anaemia of chronic disorders*‡ (p. 90)

Sideroblastic anaemias*

Lead poisoning*

Heterozygosity and homozygosity for β-thalassaemia† (p. 63)

α⁺-thalassaemia trait†‡ (p. 62)

α⁰-thalassaemia trait† (p. 62)

HbH disease† (p. 62)

Heterozygotes and homozygotes for HbE† (p. 59)

Homozygotes for HbC†‡ (p. 59)

* The hypochromia is caused by impaired haem synthesis.
† The hypochromia is caused by impaired globin chain synthesis.
‡ Some patients have normochromic normocytic red cells.

Table 4.3

DIFFERENTIAL DIAGNOSIS

Investigation	Iron-deficiency anaemia	Anaemia of chronic disorders	Thalassaemia trait
Serum iron	Low	Low	Normal
Serum transferrin	Increased or normal	Decreased or normal	Normal
Serum ferritin	Decreased	Normal or increased	Normal
Marrow iron stores	Absent	Normal or increased	Normal or increased

Table 4.4 Investigations useful in distinguishing between three important causes of hypochromic microcytes.

concentrations in the serum of iron, transferrin and ferritin, and the quantity of stainable iron within bone marrow macrophages.

ANAEMIA OF CHRONIC DISORDERS

A common type of anaemia seen in hospital in-patients is that associated with chronic disorders such as chronic infections (e.g. tuberculosis), neoplasia and rheumatoid arthritis (Cartwright & Lee 1971; Sears 1992). The anaemia is primarily the result of the underproduction of red cells; there is also a mild to moderate reduction in red-cell life-span. The red cells are most often normocytic and normochromic, although in 30–35% of patients they are hypochromic and microcytic. The anaemia usually develops within the first 2 months of the disease and then stabilizes at a fairly constant level.

There are alterations in iron metabolism and it is necessary to determine whether the changes are entirely due to the chronic disorder or whether iron deficiency is also present. In both conditions, the serum iron concentration is low but the two can be distinguished by serum ferritin and transferrin measurements (Table 4.4); iron deficiency is characterized by a low serum ferritin and high transferrin whereas by contrast in the anaemia of chronic disorders, the ferritin is normal or high and the transferrin frequently low. In addition, if the MCV is below 70 fl, iron deficiency is much more likely to be present. Analysis of all three values gave complete correlation with the assessment based on bone marrow aspiration in a series of rheumatoid arthritis patients (Vreugdenhil et al. 1990). If the diagnosis from the peripheral blood tests is still in doubt, the presence or absence of storage iron in the marrow can be determined. Characteristically, iron stores are normal or increased in the anaemia of chronic disorders and absent in iron-deficiency anaemia.

The causes of the anaemia associated with chronic diseases are still in dispute, but impaired release of iron from macrophages; low erythropoietin levels for the degree of anaemia (Krantz 1994); suppression of erythropoiesis by inhibitory cytokines (tumour necrosis factor and interleukin-1 (produced by activated macrophages) and γ-interferon); and the 'stealing' of iron from transferrin by neutrophil-derived lactoferrin have been incriminated.

SIDEROBLASTIC ANAEMIAS

The term 'sideroblastic erythropoiesis' is used to describe an abnormal type of red-cell production in which a substantial proportion of erythroblasts contain a perinuclear ring of coarse iron-containing granules (Fig. 4.5, Plate 19). These granules are not usually apparent in Romanowsky-stained marrow smears but appear blue in smears stained by Perls' acid ferrocyanide method for haemosiderin. The abnormal cells are described as ring sideroblasts. Ultrastructural studies have shown that the granules within ring sideroblasts consist of iron-laden mitochondria; the iron-containing material is deposited in between the mitochondrial cristae

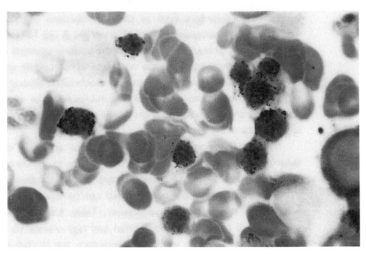

Fig. 4.5 Marrow smear from a patient with primary acquired sideroblastic anaemia, stained by Perls' acid ferrocyanide method (Prussian blue reaction). The erythroblasts contain several coarse (blue-black) iron-containing granules which are often arranged around the nucleus.

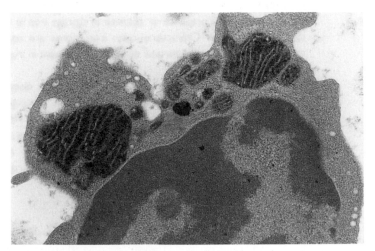

Fig. 4.6 Electron micrograph of part of a ring sideroblast showing very electron-dense material between the cristae of enlarged mitochondria.

(Fig. 4.6). As a result of the mitochondrial damage, a variable proportion of the red cells produced are microcytic and hypochromic.

Sideroblastic erythropoiesis may be found both as an inherited (usually X-linked recessive) and an acquired condition. The abnormality occurs as an acquired condition in the myelodysplastic syndrome (p. 175) known as refractory anaemia with ring sideroblasts (primary acquired sideroblastic anaemia), and in occasional patients with chronic mye-loproliferative disorders. Acquired sideroblastic anaemia may also be secondary to excessive alcohol consumption, therapy with certain drugs (e.g. isoniazid or chloramphenicol), and lead poisoning.

Iron overload

As the body has no mechanism for actively increasing iron excretion, a progressive increase in total body iron stores occurs in two categories of patients. There are those who absorb increased quantities of iron over a prolonged period, and those who receive repeated blood transfusions over several years for conditions such as thalassaemia major, aplastic anaemia and red-cell aplasia. Iron absorption from a normal diet is inappropriately increased from birth in the condition known as idiopathic haemochromatosis which is inherited as an autosomal recessive trait. Homozygotes usually develop symptoms from tissue damage due to severe iron overload between the ages of 40 and 60 years. Iron absorp-tion is also increased in patients with severe erythroid hyperplasia due to peripheral haemolysis or ineffectiveness of erythropoiesis. Some patients in the latter category (e.g. with thalassaemia intermedia or inherited sideroblastic anaemia) may have iron overload even when they have not been transfused to any significant extent.

When the iron stores become greatly increased (Plate 20), the heart, liver, endocrine organs and other tissues undergo progressive damage. Clinicopathological manifestations of severe iron overload include a bronze skin pigmentation, cardiac dysfunction, cirrhosis, diabetes mellitus, testicular atrophy and arthropathy.

The serum ferritin level is the most useful screening test for iron overload and may be as high as 10 000 µg/l in severely affected patients. It is a poor guide to the amount of iron overload, particularly when ferritin values exceed 4000 µg/l. The diagnosis of iron overload should therefore be confirmed by liver biopsy which permits both the chemical estimation of the quantity of iron in the tissue and a histological assess-ment of the distribution of haemosiderin and the extent of tissue damage. High serum ferritin levels may be found in the presence of normal iron stores in conditions such as malignancy, infection and hepatocellular damage.

Idiopathic haemochromatosis is treated by repeated phlebotomy. Iron overload secondary to blood transfusion should be prevented or limited by the administration of the iron chelator desferrioxamine (p. 65).

Patients who are developing iron overload secondary to increased erythropoietic activity should also be treated with desferrioxamine.

References

Berry W.T.C., Nash F.A. (1954) Symptoms as a guide to anaemia. *Br. Med. J.* **1**, 918.

Beutler E. (1959) Red cell indices in the diagnosis of iron deficiency anaemia. *Ann. Intern. Med.* **50**, 313–322.

Beveridge B.R., Bannerman R.M., Evanson J.M., Witts L.J. (1965) Hypochromic anaemia. A retrospective study and follow-up of 378 in-patients. *Q. J. Med.* **34**, 145–161.

Burman D. (1982) Iron deficiency in infancy and childhood. *Clin. Haematol.* **11**, 339–351.

Cartwright G.E., Lee G.R. (1971) The anaemia of chronic disorders. Annotation. *Br. J. Haematol.* **21**, 147–152.

Colomer J., Colomer C., Gutierrez D., Jubert A., Nolasco A., Donat J., Fernandez Delgado R., Donat F., Alvarez Dardet C. (1990) Anaemia during pregnancy as a risk factor for infant iron deficiency. *Paediatr. Perinat. Epidemiol.* **4**, 196–204.

Cook J.D., Skikne B.S., Baynes R.D. (1993) Serum transferrin receptor. *Ann. Rev. Med.* **44**, 63–74.

Crampton P., Farrell A., Tuohy P. (1994) Iron deficiency anaemia in infants. *N. Z. Med. J.* **107**, 60–61.

Dallman P.R. (1989) Iron deficiency: does it matter? *J. Intern. Med.* **226**, 365–372.

Duggan M.B., Steel G., Elwys G., Harbottle L., Noble C. (1991) Iron status, energy intake, and nutritional status of healthy young Asian children. *Arch. Dis. Child.* **66**, 1386–1389.

Godel J.C., Pabst H.F., Hodges P.E., Johnson K.E. (1992) Iron status and pregnancy in a Northern Canadian population: Relationship to diet and iron supplementation. *Can. J. Public Health* **83**, 339–343.

Hallberg L., Hoogdaht A.M., Nilsson L., Rybo G. (1966) Menstrual blood loss and iron deficiency. *Acta Med. Scand.* **180**, 639–650.

Hallberg L., Bengtsson C., Lapidus L., Lindstedt G., Lundberg P.A., Hulten L. (1993a) Screening for iron deficiency: An analysis based on bone-marrow examinations and serum ferritin determinations in a population sample of women. *Br. J. Haematol.* **85**, 787–798.

Hallberg L., Hulten L., Lindstedt G., Lundbert P.A., Mark A., Purens J., Svanberg B.S., Wolin B. (1993b) Prevalence of iron deficiency in Swedish adolescents. *Pediatr. Res.* **34**, 680–687.

Hammond J., Chinn S., Richardson H., Rona R. (1994) Serum total cholesterol and ferritin and blood haemoglobin concentrations in primary schoolchildren. *Arch. Dis. Child.* **70**, 373–375.

Holt J.M., Gear M.W.L., Warner G.T. (1970) The role of chronic blood loss in the pathogenesis of postgastrectomy iron-deficiency anaemia. *Gut* **11**, 847–850.

Jacobs A., Kilpatrick G.S., Withey J.L. (1965) Iron-deficiency anaemia in adults, prevalence and prevention. *Postgrad. Med. J.* **41**, 418–424.

Joosten E., Dereymaeker L., Pelemans W., Hiele M. (1993) Significance of a low serum ferritin level in elderly in-patients. *Postgrad. Med. J.* **69**, 397–400.

Krantz S.B. (1994) Pathogenesis and treatment of the anemia of chronic disease. *Am. J. Med. Sci.* **307**, 353–359.

Mills A.F. (1990) Surveillance for anaemia: Risk factors in patterns of milk intake. *Arch. Dis. Child.* **65**, 428–431.

Milman N., Kirchhoff M. (1991) Iron stores in 1433, 30- to 60-year old Danish males. Evaluation by serum ferritin and haemoglobin. *Scand. J. Clin. Lab. Invest.* **517**, 635–641.

Milman N., Rosdahl N., Lyhne N., Jorgensen T., Graudal N. (1993) Iron status in Danish women aged 35–65 years. Relation to menstruation and method of contraception. *Acta Obstet. Gynecol. Scand.* **72**, 601–605.

Milman N., Agger A.O., Nielsen O.J. (1994) Iron status markers and serum erythropoietin in 120 mothers and newborn infants. Effect of iron supplementation in normal pregnancy. *Acta Obstet. Gynecol. Scand.* **73**, 200–204.

Newton M., Mosey L.M., Egii G.E., Gifford W.B., Hull C.T. (1961) Blood loss during and immediately after delivery. *Obstet. Gynecol.* **17**, 9–18.

Parks Y.A., Wharton B.A. (1989) Iron deficiency and the brain. *Acta Paediatr. Scand.* **361**, Suppl. **78**, 71–77.

Rockey D.C., Cello J.P. (1993) Evaluation of the gastrointestinal tract in patients with iron-deficiency anemia. *N. Engl. J. Med.* **329**, 1691–1695.

Sears D.A. (1992) Anemia of chronic disease. *Med. Clin. North. Am.* **76**, 567–579.

Sheard N.F. (1994) Iron deficiency and infant development. *Nutr. Rev.* **52**, 137–140.

Tovey F.I., Godfrey J.E., Lewin M.R. (1990) A gastrectomy population: 25–30 years on. *Postgrad. Med. J.* **66**, 450–456.

Vreugdenhil G., Baltus C.A.M., Van Eijk H.G., Swaak A.J.G. (1990) Anaemia of chronic disease: Diagnostic significance of erythrocyte and serological parameters in iron deficient rheumatoid arthritis patients. *Br. J. Rheumatol.* **29**, 105–110.

Review

Hershko C. (ed.) (1994) *Clinical Disorders of Iron Metabolism.* Baillières Clinical Haematology, International Practice and Research, Vol 7/No 4. Baillière Tindall, London.

CHAPTER 5

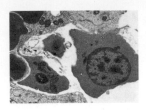

Macrocytosis and Macrocytic Anaemia

Objectives in learning

1 To understand the relationship between the terms macrocytic, megaloblastic, vitamin B_{12} deficiency and folate deficiency.

2 To know the dietary sources, mechanisms of absorption, extent and site of storage, and the mechanism and rate of loss from the body of both B_{12} and folate.

3 To be aware of the causes of B_{12} deficiency and of folate deficiency.

4 To know the symptoms and signs of B_{12} deficiency referable to the gastrointestinal tract, central nervous system, peripheral nerves, and the cardiovascular and haematological systems.

5 To understand the principles involved in making the diagnosis of pernicious anaemia from various laboratory investigations.

6 To understand the method of differentiation of megaloblastic anaemia due to B_{12} deficiency from that due to folate deficiency.

7 To understand the principles of treatment with both B_{12} and folate.

8 To know the B_{12}- and folate-independent causes of macrocytosis.

Macrocytosis and macrocytic anaemia may be found in a variety of unrelated diseases. In some conditions associated with macrocytosis, the red-cell precursors have a normal morphology (i.e. there is normoblastic erythropoiesis) and in others they show morphological abnormalities of the type seen in vitamin B_{12} deficiency caused by pernicious anaemia. Marrows containing such abnormal erythroblasts are described as displaying megaloblastic erythropoiesis. During the investigation of the cause of a macrocytic anaemia it is often helpful to determine the type of erythropoiesis by examining stained smears of bone marrow cells obtained by aspiration biopsy.

Megaloblastic erythropoiesis

The causes of megaloblastic erythropoiesis are:

1 a deficiency of vitamin B_{12} or folate;

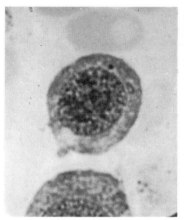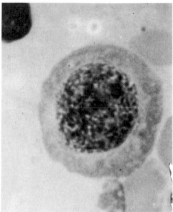

Fig. 5.1 Early polychromatic megaloblasts from a patient with severe pernicious anaemia. These cells are larger and have smaller granules of condensed nuclear chromatin than the two early polychromatic normoblasts in Fig. 1.7c on p. 15.

2 disturbances of vitamin B_{12} or folate metabolism (e.g. caused by nitrous oxide or methotrexate), and

3 biochemical abnormalities unrelated to vitamin B_{12} or folate (e.g. orotic aciduria; therapy with antipurines).

Megaloblastic erythropoiesis is characterized by abnormal red-cell precursors known as megaloblasts, in which cell and nuclear diameters are larger than in normal red-cell precursors (normoblasts) and in which the condensed nuclear chromatin is more finely dispersed than in normoblasts of corresponding cytoplasmic maturity (Fig. 5.1, Plates 21, 22). Marrows showing megaloblastic erythropoiesis also frequently contain giant metamyelocytes. These are about twice the size of normal metamyelocytes and have horse-shoe-shaped or long, twisted, ribbon-like nuclei (Fig. 5.2).

Megaloblasts suffer from a gross disturbance of cell proliferation, and many of the more mature megaloblasts are ingested and degraded by bone marrow macrophages (Fig. 5.3). Thus, despite the fact that megaloblastic marrows show erythroid hyperplasia, this increased ineffectiveness of erythropoiesis (p. 17) results in the rate of delivery of new red cells into the circulation being suboptimal for the degree of anaemia. Many of the giant metamyelocytes are also destroyed within the marrow (ineffective granulocytopoiesis) (Wickramasinghe 1972).

Megaloblastic changes occur when DNA synthesis is disordered, but the detailed biochemical basis of the morphological abnormality remains

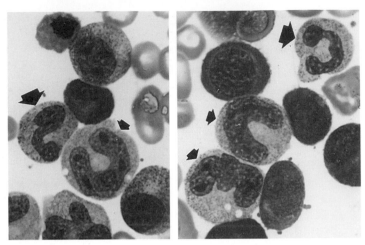

Fig. 5.2 Giant metamyelocytes (small arrows) near normal-sized metamyelocytes (large arrows) in a marrow smear from a patient with untreated pernicious anaemia. One of the giant metamyelocytes has an E-shaped nucleus.

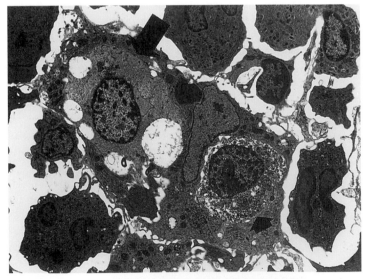

Fig. 5.3 Electron micrograph of a bone marrow macrophage from a patient with severe pernicious anaemia. The cytoplasm of the macrophage contains two ingested megaloblasts (arrowed) at various stages of degradation.

uncertain. The ways in which vitamin B_{12} and folate deficiency may impair DNA synthesis are discussed later (pp. 102–104 and p. 114)

In vitamin B_{12} and folate deficiency, megaloblastic changes are not confined to bone marrow cells; the characteristic nuclear abnormality is found in a variety of epithelial cells, including those of the buccal and nasal mucosa, tongue, urinary tract, jejunum, vagina and cervix uteri.

Blood picture in patients with megaloblastic haemopoiesis

In many patients there is a high mean cell volume (MCV) associated with varying degrees of anaemia. Some patients have a high MCV without anaemia. However, even in these the haemoglobin (Hb) level may rise following the correction of the underlying defect indicating that their Hb at presentation, although within the normal range, was below their own normal value. The absolute reticulocyte count is variable, being either reduced, normal or slightly increased. Any increase is much less than that seen in an individual with normally functioning bone marrow and a similar degree of anaemia. Red-cell life-span is slightly decreased. The anaemia is mainly due to the ineffectiveness of megaloblastic erythropoiesis. The blood films of patients with megaloblastic erythropoiesis contain macrocytes, some of which are oval in shape (Fig. 5.4, Plate 48). The red cells also show anisocytosis and poikilocytosis, particularly in moderately and severely anaemic cases. Macrocytic anaemias caused by megaloblastic haemopoiesis are referred to as megaloblastic anaemias.

In patients with vitamin B_{12}- or folate-related megaloblastic hae-mopoiesis, the circulating neutrophil granulocytes frequently show hypersegmentation of their nuclei (Fig. 5.5, Plate 48). Under normal circumstances, 3% or less of neutrophil granulocytes have five or more nuclear segments, but in vitamin B_{12} or folic-acid deficiency more than 3% are hypersegmented and there may even be occasional cells with eight to ten segments. Hypersegmentation is not diagnostic of vitamin B_{12} or folate deficiency; it may also occur in anaemia due to iron deficiency and in renal failure, even when B_{12} and folate stores are adequate. Hypersegmented neutrophil polymorphs are not derived from giant metamyelocytes but from normal-looking metamyelocytes. When the megaloblastic changes caused by vitamin B_{12} or folate deficiency are severe, there may be neutropenia and thrombocytopenia (due to ineffec-tive granulocytopoiesis and thrombocytopoiesis).

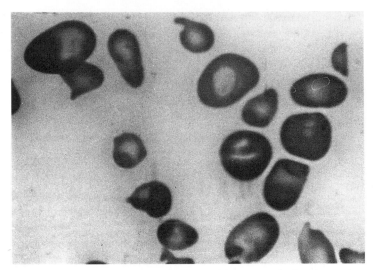

Fig. 5.4 Blood film from a patient with pernicious anaemia showing oval macrocytes and other poikilocytes.

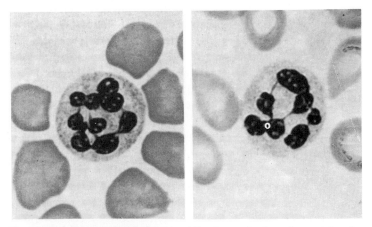

Fig. 5.5 Two hypersegmented neutrophil polymorphs from the peripheral blood smear of a patient with vitamin B$_{12}$ deficiency due to pernicious anaemia.

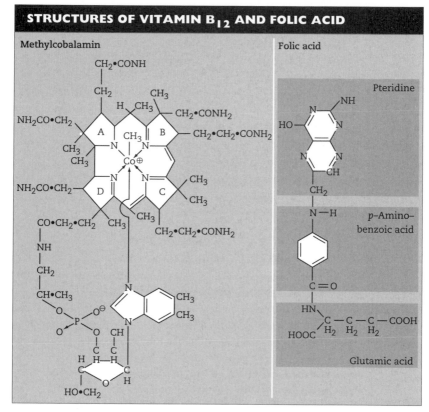

STRUCTURES OF VITAMIN B₁₂ AND FOLIC ACID

Methylcobalamin

Folic acid

Fig. 5.6 The structure of vitamin B₁₂ and folic acid.

Megaloblastic anaemias (macrocytic anaemias with megaloblastic erythropoiesis)

VITAMIN B₁₂ DEFICIENCY

Biochemistry

The B_{12} molecule is composed of: (a) a planar corrin nucleus made up of four pyrrole rings (A–D); (b) the ribonucleotide of 5,6-dimethyl-benzimidazole; and (c) a cobalt atom situated at the centre of the corrin nucleus which is coordinately bonded to the four pyrrole rings, one of the nitrogen atoms of the ribonucleotide and to an organic group (Fig. 5.6). In the two biologically active forms of vitamin B_{12}, namely methylcobalamin and adenosylcobalamin, the organic group bound to the cobalt atom is methyl and adenosyl, respectively. The biochemical mechanisms underlying the anaemia and neuropathy of vitamin B_{12} deficiency are still uncertain. However, both the anaemia and neuropathy may be caused by an impairment of one of the two reactions known to require vitamin B_{12} in man, namely the methylation of homocysteine to methionine by homocysteine methyltransferase, which is dependent both on 5-methyltetrahydrofolate (p. 114) and methylcobalamin.

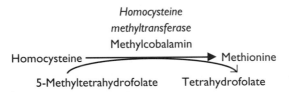

Since the 5-methyltetrahydrofolate serves as the methyl donor, failure of this reaction results not only in impaired methionine synthesis but also in the accumulation of 5-methyltetrahydrofolate and homocysteine, with increased concentrations of homocysteine in the serum. Impairment of the homocysteine methyltransferase reaction eventually leads to a reduction in the availability of 5,10-methylenetetrahydrofolate for the methylation of deoxyuridine monophosphate to thymidine monophosphate and, consequently, to reduced synthesis of thymidine triphosphate (Fig. 5.7). This, in turn, causes: (a) slowing of DNA strand elongation due to an inadequate supply of thymidine triphosphate for DNA synthesis; (b) accumulation of deoxyuridine monophosphate within the cell and its phosphorylation to deoxyuridine triphosphate; and (c) misincorporation into DNA of uracil (from deoxyuridine triphosphate) in lieu of thymine (Fig. 5.7). Although there is little doubt that DNA synthesis is impaired in B_{12} deficiency, the critical defect underlying the megaloblastic change remains unclear.

It has been proposed that impairment of the homocysteine methyltransferase reaction results in reduced levels of 5,10-methylenetetrahydrofolate by the trapping of intracellular folates in the form of 5-methyltetrahydrofolate which cannot be converted to 5,10-methylenetetrahydrofolate (methylfolate trap hypothesis). However, recent data suggest that the important consequence of the impairment of the homocysteine methyltransferase reaction is not the intra-cellular accumulation of 5-methyltetrahydrofolate but the failure of methionine synthesis which in turn results in reduced synthesis of

Continued

S-adenosylmethionine and, consequently, a decreased supply of active formate required for the synthesis of 5,10-methylenetetrahydrofolate (formate starvation hypothesis) (Chanarin et al. 1980).

The second of the two reactions known to require B_{12} in humans is the adenosylcobalamin-dependent conversion of methylmalonyl CoA to succinyl CoA by the enzyme methylmalonyl CoA mutase.

$$\text{Propionyl CoA} \longrightarrow \text{Methylmalonyl CoA} \xrightarrow{\text{Adenosyl } B_{12}} \text{Succinyl CoA}$$
$$\textit{Methylmalonyl CoA mutase}$$

The involvement of B_{12} in this reaction explains the finding of raised serum methylmalonic acid concentrations in B_{12} deficiency.

There is some evidence that the neuropathy associated with B_{12} deficiency may be caused by hypomethylation of nervous system proteins due to reduced availability of S-adenosylmethionine. Whether impairment of the adenosylcobalamin-dependent conversion of methylmalonyl CoA to succinyl CoA is also involved in the pathogenesis of the neuropathy is controversial.

Vitamin B_{12} in the diet

Vitamin B_{12} is produced entirely by bacteria and none is present in plants. Herbivores obtain vitamin B_{12} mainly as a result of synthesis by bacteria in their rumen; other animals and man obtain it by eating food of animal origin. The average amount of B_{12} in a mixed diet is about $5\,\mu g$/day.

Mechanism of absorption

The B_{12} in food is largely protein-bound and is released from its bound state within the stomach by the action of pepsin. Most of the released B_{12} binds immediately to R-binder (a B_{12}-binding protein found in saliva and gastric juice). The B_{12} is released from the B_{12}–R-binder complex in the jejunum by the action of pancreatic trypsin; the released B_{12} then binds to intrinsic factor. The function of intrinsic factor is to transport B_{12} into the epithelial cells of the distal half of the small intestine.

Intrinsic factor is produced in the body and fundus of the stomach by the same cells that produce hydrochloric acid, namely, the gastric parietal cells. It is a glycoprotein with a molecular weight of about 57 kD and each molecule binds one molecule of B_{12}. The amount of intrinsic factor in the gastric juice can be estimated indirectly by measuring the amount of vitamin B_{12} that it can bind. The average basal secretion of 3000 units per hour increases three to five-fold after the administration of stimulants such as histamine and gastrin. The quantity of vitamin B_{12} required to be absorbed daily to maintain body stores is about 1–3 μg, and only

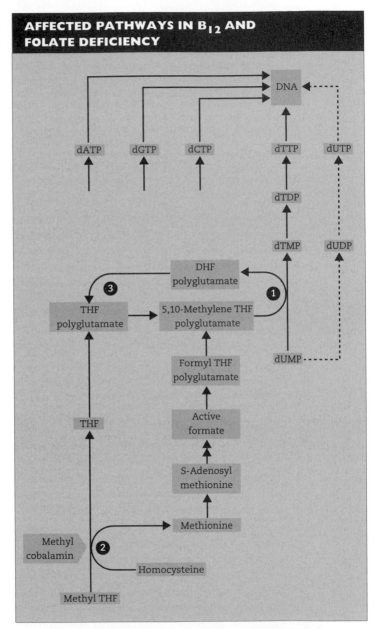

Fig. 5.7 Biochemical pathways affected in B_{12} and folate deficiency. dUMP, Deoxyuridine monophosphate; dTMP, Deoxythymidine monophosphate; dTTP, Deoxythymidine triphosphate; dUTP, Deoxyuridine triphosphate; THF, Tetrahydrofolate. Enzymes: (1) thymidylate synthase, (2) homocysteine methyltransferase (methionine synthase), (3) dihydrofolate reductase.

1000–3000 units of intrinsic factor are necessary for its absorption. Thus, the amount of intrinsic factor produced daily is considerably in excess of that required for vitamin B_{12} absorption (Ardeman & Chanarin 1965). The minimum quantity of B_{12} that must be absorbed daily to maintain health (rather than to maintain body stores) may be less than $0.5\,\mu g$.

Storage and rate of loss of vitamin B_{12}

Vitamin B_{12} is mainly stored in the liver and the average healthy adult has a total body content of 3–5 mg. Loss of vitamin B_{12} takes place in the urine and faeces mainly through desquamation of epithelial cells and through excretion in the bile.

The rate of loss of vitamin B_{12} is approximately 0.05–0.1% of the body content each day. There is therefore a delay of 2 years or more between the appearance of a lesion leading to impaired absorption of B_{12} and the reduction of the B_{12} store to a level (possibly about 300–500 μg) which causes megaloblastic anaemia. For instance, following the abrupt cessation of B_{12} absorption as a consequence of total gastrectomy, it takes about 2–10 years before megaloblastic anaemia develops.

VITAMIN B_{12} NEUROPATHY

Patients with vitamin B_{12} deficiency due to any cause may develop degenerative changes in the nervous system (Pant et al. 1968). The pathological changes are often considered under three headings:

1 peripheral neuropathy;
2 subacute combined degeneration of the cord, and
3 focal demyelinization of the white matter of the brain.

In subacute combined degeneration of the cord there is patchy degeneration of the posterior and lateral columns which is most marked in (but not confined to) the lower cervical and upper thoracic segments (Fig. 5.8). Histologically, the degenerating areas contain empty spaces which are surrounded by myelin-laden macrophages. The term 'subacute combined degeneration' of the cord is, however, misleading since the onset of symptoms is usually insidious and not subacute, lesions of the posterior and lateral columns can occur alone and are not necessarily combined, and the syndrome frequently includes lesions of the peripheral nerves or cerebral hemispheres as well as the spinal cord.

Symptoms and signs usually affect the lower limbs first and are symmetrical (Healton et al. 1991). The commonest symptoms are paraesthesia in the extremities, ataxia of gait and muscle weakness. Others include poor vision, orthostatic dizziness, stiffness of the limbs, impotence and impairment of bladder and rectal control. Some impairment of memory, irritability, mild depression, apathy and fluctuations of

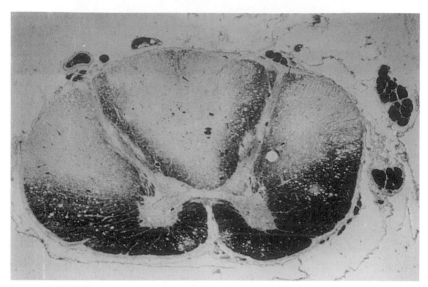

Fig. 5.8 Subacute combined degeneration of the cervical spinal cord. The posterior and lateral columns show demyelination and, therefore, appear pale (Weigert–Pal method for myelin). (Reproduced with permission from Dr R.O. Barnard.)

mood are relatively common but serious psychiatric symptoms, (e.g. stupor, hallucinations, paranoia, severe depression and manic psychosis) are uncommon. However, occasional patients have been rescued from psychiatric institutions and restored to health by B_{12} injections. Blindness due to optic atrophy has been reported but is rare.

On the basis of a clinical examination of the nervous system, it is sometimes difficult to distinguish between peripheral neuritis and posterior column involvement, since in both conditions tendon reflexes and vibrational and positional sense may be reduced, and ataxia may be present. However, hyperalgesia of calf muscles favours peripheral neuritis, whereas a disproportionate reduction in positional and vibrational sense up to the pelvis compared to touch and pin-prick favours involvement of the lateral columns. An extensor plantar response indicates pyramidal tract involvement. Individual patients vary as to the extent to which lesions in the posterior columns, lateral columns, or peripheral nerves dominate the neurological syndrome. Spinal cord lesions may occur in the absence of peripheral neuritis and vice versa.

Neurological involvement may occur without anaemia although the bone marrow usually shows mild megaloblastic changes.

VITAMIN B$_{12}$ DEFICIENCY

Inadequate intake
Veganism

Inadequate secretion of intrinsic factor
Pernicious anaemia
Total or partial gastrectomy
Congenital intrinsic factor deficiency (rare)

Inadequate release of B$_{12}$ from food
Partial gastrectomy, vagotomy, gastric dysfunction

Diversion of dietary B$_{12}$
Abnormal intestinal bacterial flora
  Multiple jejunal diverticula, small intestinal strictures, stagnant
  intestinal loops
Diphyllobothrium latum

Malabsorption
Crohn's disease, ileal resection, chronic tropical sprue, congenital
  selective B$_{12}$ malabsorption with proteinuria (Imerslund–Gräsbeck
  syndrome)

Table 5.1 Mechanisms and causes of vitamin B$_{12}$ deficiency.

CAUSES OF VITAMIN B$_{12}$ DEFICIENCY

These are summarized in Table 5.1. The two most common mechanisms of vitamin B$_{12}$ deficiency are a failure to secrete intrinsic factor and a failure to absorb vitamin B$_{12}$ as a result of abnormalities in the distal ileum.

Inadequate intake

Veganism

Vitamin B$_{12}$ deficiency resulting from a very low B$_{12}$ content in the diet only occurs in strict vegetarians who eat no animal protein at all (vegans). Although there is no vitamin B$_{12}$ in plants, the vegan diet probably contains some B$_{12}$ as a result of bacterial contamination of water and vegetables and bacterial fermentation of bruised vegetables. Low serum vitamin B$_{12}$ levels are found in over 50% of vegans. However, most vegans with low serum B$_{12}$ levels are healthy and do not show anaemia or macrocytosis; only a minority suffer from megaloblastic anaemia or vitamin B$_{12}$ neuropathy.

Inadequate secretion of intrinsic factor

Pernicious anaemia

Aetiology and pathogenesis
Pernicious anaemia is a condition in which the absorption of vitamin B_{12} is greatly impaired due to a failure or marked reduction of intrinsic factor secretion secondary to severe atrophic gastritis or gastric atrophy. The basal secretion of intrinsic factor is reduced to only 0–200 units per hour and is unaffected by stimulants such as histamine. Vitamin B_{12} deficiency develops and leads to megaloblastic anaemia, neurological damage, or both. One of the first descriptions of this condition was by Thomas Addison of Guy's Hospital, London, in 1849, and the disease is therefore sometimes referred to as Addisonian pernicious anaemia. About 20% of patients have a relative with pernicious anaemia, indicating that genetic factors may predispose to the development of gastric atrophy in adult life. Furthermore, 10% of patients with pernicious anaemia have clinical or subclinical autoimmune thyroid disease suggesting that the gastric atrophy has an autoimmune basis. Antibodies against gastric parietal cells are found in the serum in about 85% of patients with pernicious anaemia; these are directed against the α and β subunits of the proton pump (H^+, K^+ ATPase) of the gastric parietal cell (Glesson & Toh 1991). Antibodies against intrinsic factor are found in the serum of about 55% of patients and in the gastric juice of about 60%. However, the fact that antibodies cannot be detected in all cases, combined with the observation that a few patients with thyroid disorders have anti-intrinsic factor antibodies in their serum but do not have B_{12} deficiency, suggest that these antibodies are not the primary cause of the gastric atrophy and the resulting failure of intrinsic factor secretion; they may instead be a consequence of the damage to the gastric mucosa. It is possible on the other hand that the gastric atrophy is the result of cell-mediated immune reactions against parietal and other gastric cells as is the case in a murine model of autoimmune chronic atrophic gastritis (Glesson & Toh 1991).

All cases of pernicious anaemia have a gastric lesion, varying from severe atrophic gastritis to gastric atrophy. As both intrinsic factor and hydrochloric acid are produced by the same cell (i.e. the parietal cell), histamine-fast and pentagastrin-fast achlorhydria is an invariable accompaniment of pernicious anaemia and the diagnosis cannot be made if appreciable quantities of hydrochloric acid are found to be secreted. The pH of resting gastric juice in pernicious anaemia is between 6 and 8 and after maximal stimulation with histamine or pentagastrin it does not fall by more than 0.5 pH units.

However, not all individuals with gastric atrophy or achlorhydria have pernicious anaemia, presumably because many individuals with these abnormalities continue to secrete the small quantities of intrinsic factor required for the absorption of adequate amounts of B_{12}.

Pernicious anaemia should not be regarded merely as a condition in which there is a deficient production of red cells and damage to the nervous system, but rather as a vitamin deficiency disease affecting many cell types in the body, including all dividing cells. Symptoms and signs are referable not only to the blood and neural tissue (brain, spinal cord, peripheral nerves), but also to the gastrointestinal tract (from the tongue down to the colon), skin and other tissues and organs (e.g. ovaries). Severe anaemia may aggravate co-existing cardiac disease.

Clinical features
Pernicious anaemia is most common in people of northern European extraction and in England its prevalence is about 1 per 1000 of the population. Only 10% of cases are diagnosed under 40 years of age; the prevalence increases with age, reaching about 0.5% between the ages of 70 and 79 years. Females are one and a half times more frequently affected than males.

Symptoms develop slowly. Common presenting symptoms are tiredness and weakness, dyspnoea, paraesthesia, sore tongue, vague gastrointestinal disturbance (anorexia, nausea, vomiting, dyspepsia, constipation or diarrhoea) and loss of weight. Other symptoms include subfertility and, rarely, hyperpigmentation of the skin of the hands. Various neurological and psychiatric symptoms may develop in a proportion of cases, due to a vitamin B_{12} neuropathy (p. 105). Apart from pallor, the most frequent sign is atrophic glossitis. Commonly, some degree of papillary atrophy of the tongue is seen as an unusual smoothness at the edges, but this sometimes spreads over the entire dorsal surface (Fig. 5.9). Occasionally, the tongue is red, painful and ulcerated. Fever may be present when the anaemia is severe. The spleen is palpable in some cases. Male patients with pernicious anaemia have an increased incidence of gastric carcinoma.

Haematological and biochemical changes
The haematological picture is that seen in any vitamin B_{12}- or folate-related megaloblastic anaemia (p. 99). The Hb level may be within the normal range in patients diagnosed early but decreases progressively as the degree of deficiency increases. The blood count shows a high

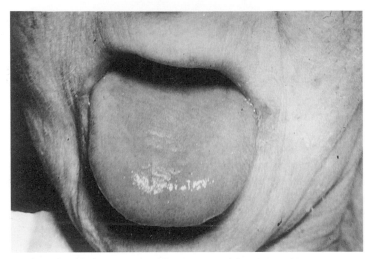

Fig. 5.9 Glossitis in a woman with severe pernicious anaemia.

MCV provided that the pernicious anaemia is not complicated by co-existing conditions such as iron deficiency or thalassaemia trait. The marrow is hypercellular and in severely anaemic patients virtually all of the fat cells of the marrow are replaced by haemopoietic cells. Haemopoiesis is megaloblastic in type (p. 97) and giant metamyelocytes may be present.

There may be a slight increase in the serum bilirubin level and an increase in serum lactate dehydrogenase; these changes result mainly from the intramedullary destruction of erythroblasts and partly from a mild degree of peripheral haemolysis. The level of B_{12} in the serum is virtually always reduced. However, low serum B_{12} levels should be considered as presumptive rather than definitive evidence of B_{12} deficiency, since they are also found in the absence of any other evidence of B_{12} deficiency, in one-third of folate-deficient patients and in some pregnant women. About 60% of patients with pernicious anaemia have low red-cell folate levels and the remainder have normal levels. The concentrations of both methylmalonic acid and homocysteine in the serum are raised in virtually all patients (Stabler et al. 1990).

Diagnosis (see Table 5.2 on p. 115)
In order to establish the diagnosis of pernicious anaemia, it is necessary to demonstrate either a marked reduction or the absence of intrinsic factor in gastric juice. This is usually done indirectly by performing a Schilling test (Schilling 1953). This test measures the ability of an indi-

vidual to absorb orally administered cyanocobalamin. It involves giving 1 µg of ^{57}Co-cyanocobalamin by mouth and, at the same time, 1 mg of non-radioactive cyanocobalamin intramuscularly. The urine passed over the next 24 hours is collected and its radioactivity determined. The large intramuscular dose of non-radioactive B_{12} saturates the B_{12}-binding proteins in the plasma and thus causes a substantial proportion of any absorbed ^{57}Co-B_{12} to be excreted in the urine. B_{12} absorption is considered to be impaired when the urinary excretion of ^{57}Co-B_{12} over the 24 hours is less than 10% of the dose given by mouth. In pernicious anaemia it is often below 5%. If the test is abnormal it should be repeated giving both intrinsic factor and ^{57}Co-B_{12} by mouth; if the low B_{12} absorption in the patient is the result of intrinsic factor deficiency, then the absorption will be improved (but not restored to normal). This test clearly gives essential information concerning the basic defect in pernicious anaemia and is the most important of all the tests that can be performed. The diagnosis of pernicious anaemia can be more directly established by assay of intrinsic factor secretion in gastric juice but this procedure has been replaced by the simpler Schilling test and is no longer in routine use.

Treatment

Patients with pernicious anaemia may be initially treated with 1 mg hydroxocobalamin intramuscularly every 2–3 weeks over a period of 3 months to replenish body stores. Maintenance therapy with injections of 1 mg hydroxocobalamin every 3 months should be continued for the rest of their lives. It is customary to start treating patients with serious neurological symptoms with 1 mg hydroxocobalamin twice a week rather than every 2–3 weeks even though there is no evidence that more frequent injections are required for the treatment of neuropathy than of anaemia. Complicating infections and congestive cardiac failure should be treated promptly. Blood transfusion should be avoided whenever possible as this may precipitate or aggravate cardiac failure. If transfusion is necessary in severely anaemic patients, this should be done cautiously under cover of diuretics, administering no more than one to two units of packed red cells slowly over 24 hours. Some clinicians prefer to perform a one to two unit partial exchange transfusion. A number of patients with severe pernicious anaemia die suddenly, presumably of cardiac arrhythmias, shortly after the start of B_{12} therapy and this has been attributed to a fall in serum potassium consequent on a movement of potassium into cells in response to therapy with B_{12}. Patients with severe pernicious anaemia should therefore be started on oral potassium supplements at the same time as the B_{12}; the potassium should be

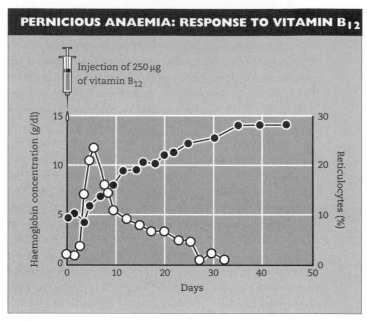

Fig. 5.10 Response of a patient with pernicious anaemia to vitamin B_{12} administration: (●) Hb concentration; (○) reticulocyte percentage.

continued for 10 days. If the cause of a severe megaloblastic anaemia is uncertain at presentation, as is often the case, treatment should be started with both hydroxocobalamin intramuscularly and folic acid orally. It must be emphasized that B_{12} deficiency should not be treated for a prolonged period with folic acid alone since, although the anaemia usually responds, neurological lesions do not and may rapidly progress.

Response to hydroxocobalamin is rapid. There is an increase in mental acuity and a sense of well-being within 24–48 hours. The reticulocyte response peaks at about 5–7 days (Fig. 5.10) and, after the first week, the Hb rises by about 1 g/week. Neurological symptoms of recent onset (less than about 3 months duration) show marked improvement and may even disappear over the first 6–12 months of therapy. More long-standing symptoms improve to a lesser extent. Psychiatric symptoms of recent onset often disappear rapidly and completely.

Total or partial gastrectomy

Megaloblastic anaemia due to vitamin B_{12} deficiency is an invariable result of total gastrectomy and develops 2–10 years after the operation, this being the time taken to exhaust the B_{12} stores present preoperatively.

Deficiency may also develop after partial gastrectomy but usually not before 5 years have elapsed, and is due in some cases to the removal of most of the intrinsic factor-producing area of the stomach and atrophy of the remaining mucosa leading to deficiency of intrinsic factor secretion. In other cases the absorption of crystalline B_{12} in the Schilling test is normal and the B_{12} deficiency is caused not by intrinsic factor deficiency, but by a failure to release B_{12} from food (see below). The incidence of deficiency after partial gastrectomy is sufficiently high to warrant routine periodic examination of the blood in all patients. Deller and Witts (1962) investigated 285 patients with partial gastrectomy for up to 12 years following the operation and found 54 who were anaemic. In most of the patients, the anaemia was due to iron deficiency, but 5% of all the patients examined had evidence of B_{12} deficiency and two of the patients had subacute combined degeneration of the cord.

Inadequate release of B_{12} from food

Some patients who have undergone vagotomy or partial gastrectomy develop B_{12} deficiency due to impaired release of B_{12} from food as a consequence of a reduced secretion of HCl and pepsin. There is increasing evidence that unexplained low serum B_{12} levels in patients who have not been subjected to vagotomy or gastric surgery may, in about 45% of cases, also result from inadequate release of B_{12} from food (Carmel 1990). The pathogenesis of the gastric dysfunction in such cases is currently under investigation.

Diversion of dietary B_{12}

Abnormal intestinal bacterial flora ('stagnant loop syndrome')

Macrocytic anaemia often arises in patients who have anatomical abnormalities of the small gut (blind loops, fistulae, diverticulosis, anastomoses and others) which lead to stasis and bacterial overgrowth. Many strains of bacteria found in stagnant small intestinal loops can take up B_{12} and convert it to inactive cobamides, leaving none for absorption by the host. Folic acid is not affected in this way: in fact folic acid may be produced by these bacteria and, therefore, red-cell folate levels may be high. Patients with this condition give an abnormal result with the Schilling test for B_{12} absorption (both without and with intrinsic factor); the abnormality is corrected after therapy with broad-spectrum antibiotics.

Infestation with the fish tapeworm

Diversion of B_{12} in the gut can occur due to successful competition by the fish tapeworm, *Diphyllobothrium latum*, which was common in Finland, but is now becoming rare.

Malabsorption

Malabsorption of B_{12} due to disease of the terminal ileum may be seen in coeliac disease and regional ileitis, and is almost invariable in chronic tropical sprue. In the latter, B_{12} deficiency is often combined with folate deficiency. Reduced absorption of B_{12} also occurs after resection of the terminal ileum.

DIAGNOSIS OF VITAMIN B_{12} DEFICIENCY

The investigations that may be of diagnostic value in a patient suspected of suffering from vitamin B_{12} deficiency are given in Table 5.2; some of these are discussed in more detail in the preceding sections. It is occasionally difficult to reliably diagnose B_{12} deficiency in patients who may have a deficiency of both B_{12} and folate (i.e. have low concentrations of both serum B_{12} and red-cell folate) (p. 110 and 118). In these cases, it is useful to investigate the haematological response to daily injections of $2\,\mu g$ hydroxocobalamin (i.e. physiological doses of B_{12}) since a response would only occur if there is a deficiency of B_{12}.

FOLATE DEFICIENCY

Biochemistry

Folic acid (pteroylmonoglutamic acid) is composed of three portions, a pteridine nucleus, *p*-aminobenzoic acid and glutamic acid (see Fig. 5.6). This compound is not biochemically active until it is reduced first to dihydrofolic acid and then to tetrahydrofolic acid. In addition, naturally occurring forms of folate contain a single carbon unit in various states of reduction (e.g. methyl, formyl, methylene). Whereas the folate present in the serum is 5-methyltetrahydrofolate monoglutamate, intracellular folates are pteroylpolyglutamates with three to seven glutamic acid residues joined together. The active forms of folate function as coenzymes in the transfer of single carbon units in: (a) amino acid metabolism; and (b) the synthesis of purines and pyrimidines required for DNA and RNA synthesis. In particular, 5,10-methylenetetrahydrofolate is required for the methylation of deoxyuridylate to thymidylate, and an impairment of this reaction may be one of the biochemical abnormalities underlying the altered DNA synthesis and the megaloblastic change in folate deficiency (also see p. 102).

TESTS

Investigation	Findings
Blood count	High MCV*
Blood film	Oval macrocytes*, hypersegmentation of neutrophil granulocytes*
Bone marrow aspiration	Megaloblasts*, giant metamyelocytes*
Serum vitamin B$_{12}$	Low (also low in one-third of folate-deficient patients)
Red-cell folate	Normal or low
Serum methylmalonic acid	Raised
Dietary assessment	No intake of animal protein in vegans
Schilling test for B$_{12}$ absorption	Abnormal in pernicious anaemia, diseases of the terminal ileum and in the 'stagnant loop syndrome'
Barium meal and follow through	Demonstrates various lesions of the small intestine in the 'stagnant loop syndrome' and in diseases of the terminal ileum
Assay of intrinsic factor in gastric juice	Very low or absent in pernicious anaemia
Therapeutic trial of 2 µg hydroxocobalamin i.m. daily	Haematological response only in B$_{12}$ deficiency

* Also found in folate deficiency.

Table 5.2 Tests useful in establishing the diagnosis and cause of vitamin B$_{12}$ deficiency.

Folates in the diet

Folates are found in foods of both animal and plant origin. An average Western diet contains daily about 400 µg of folate. The folate content of food is markedly affected by cooking as folates are rapidly destroyed by heat. About 80% of an oral dose of 200 µg pteroylglutamic acid is absorbed; the percentage absorption of polyglutamates is somewhat lower. In an adult, the minimum quantity of folate required to be absorbed daily is about 100–200 µg. The requirement is greater during pregnancy and lactation.

Absorption

This takes place mainly in the duodenum and jejunum. The folate polyglutamates in the diet are converted to monoglutamates by the action of the enzyme folate conjugase and the monoglutamates are converted to 5-methyltetrahydrofolate monoglutamate by the intestinal epithelial cell before entering the portal blood stream.

Storage and rate of loss of folates

The hepatic store of folate is normally greater than that of vitamin B_{12}, being about 8–20 mg. Folate is lost from the body in cells shed from the skin and intestinal epithelium, and in bile, urine, sweat and saliva. Folate is also lost by intracellular catabolism. The rate of loss of folate is approximately 1–2% of the total hepatic stores per day, a rate which is 10–20 times greater than the rate of loss of B_{12}. Since the minimum amount of folate required to be absorbed per day is about 100 times greater than that of B_{12}, and because folate turns over more rapidly than B_{12}, signs of folate deficiency appear much more rapidly than those of B_{12} deficiency. Thus, Herbert (1964) found that mildly megaloblastic haemopoiesis developed 5 months after a normal person was put on a folate-deficient diet, whereas it is known that after total gastrectomy, anaemia due to B_{12} deficiency does not develop for 2 years or more.

FACTORS CAUSING FOLATE DEFICIENCY

These are summarized in Table 5.3.

Inadequate diet

Megaloblastic anaemia due to inadequate intake of folate may be seen in the poor, the elderly, the mentally disturbed, chronic alcoholics and infants fed on goats' milk which is low in folate (goats milk anaemia).

FOLATE DEFICIENCY

Inadequate dietary intake

Malabsorption
Coeliac disease, jejunal resection, tropical sprue

Increased requirement
Pregnancy, premature infants, chronic haemolytic anaemias, myelofibrosis, various malignant diseases

Table 5.3 Causes of folate deficiency.

Malabsorption

Since folate is absorbed in the upper part of the small intestine, diseases which affect this part, such as coeliac disease and tropical sprue, may cause megaloblastic anaemia due to folate deficiency. Jejunal resection may also be followed by folate deficiency. In these malabsorption syndromes, folate deficiency is commonly associated with iron deficiency. This is because iron is absorbed by the same region of the small bowel as folate.

Increased requirement

Folate deficiency and megaloblastic anaemia are found whenever there is an increased demand for folate which is not met by absorption from an adequate diet. The increased requirement for folate may result from increased nucleic acid synthesis (e.g. pregnancy and chronic haemolytic anaemia) or from increased loss of folate from the body (e.g. infection with sustained pyrexia, desquamating skin diseases such as psoriasis).

Megaloblastic anaemia of pregnancy

Before the use of folate supplements during pregnancy, macrocytic anaemia due to folate deficiency was found in 0.5–5% of all pregnancies in the UK (Giles 1966; Chanarin et al. 1968). However, examination of the bone marrow during pregnancy revealed that megaloblastic haemopoiesis was even more common, being found in about one-third of cases. The diagnosis of megaloblastic anaemia is usually made after the 36th week of gestation or during the first 4 weeks of the postpartum period. The prevalence of megaloblastic anaemia of pregnancy is much higher in developing countries than in the UK.

The chief cause of folate deficiency in pregnancy is the greatly increased DNA and RNA synthesis associated with the growth of the fetus, placenta and uterus, and the expansion of the red-cell mass of the mother. It has been calculated that folate requirements increase approximately three times during pregnancy (Chanarin et al. 1968). Several subsidiary factors also play a part. About one-third of patients have anorexia and consequently a reduced food intake (Giles 1966). There also appears to be a reduction in folate absorption during pregnancy, and an increase in folate requirement may result from urinary infection.

DIAGNOSIS OF FOLATE DEFICIENCY

The haematological features of folate deficiency are macrocytosis with or without anaemia, hypersegmentation of circulating neutrophil granulocytes and megaloblastic haemopoiesis (pp. 97–100). In order to establish that these changes are caused by folate deficiency rather than by any of the other causes of megaloblastic haemopoiesis, it is necessary to establish that the patient has reduced folate stores. This is usually done by measuring red-cell folate levels. Serum folate levels are much less reliable than red-cell folate levels in assessing folate stores as they are readily affected by a short period of negative folate balance. However, even a low red-cell folate level cannot on its own be considered proof of folate deficiency since low values are found in 60% of vitamin B_{12}-deficient patients. In practice, therefore, the diagnosis of folate deficiency requires not only the finding of a low red-cell folate level in the appropriate clinical setting, but also the exclusion of vitamin B_{12} deficiency by demonstrating a normal serum B_{12} level or a normal Schilling test in those patients with borderline or low serum vitamin B_{12} levels. Folate-deficient patients have raised serum levels of homocysteine but not of methylmalonic acid, whilst B_{12}-deficient patients have raised levels of both metabolites. However, such measurements are only made in a few specialist laboratories.

A tedious, and infrequently used, but simple method of establishing the diagnosis of folate deficiency is to demonstrate a haematological response to daily injections of physiological doses of folic acid (e.g. $200\,\mu g$ daily); no response occurs in B_{12} deficiency. It is noteworthy that pharmacological doses of folic acid (5 mg daily by mouth) cause a temporary correction of the anaemia in B_{12} deficiency. However, if folate therapy is continued for more than 3 months, the anaemia recurs and neurological damage may be precipitated.

The cause of the folate deficiency is determined by taking a detailed dietary history and by performing tests of small intestinal function (including jejunal biopsy) when appropriate.

TREATMENT OF FOLATE DEFICIENCY

In an adult, macrocytosis or megaloblastic anaemia due to folate deficiency should be treated with 5 mg folic acid daily by mouth. The duration of treatment depends on the underlying disease but should, in any case, be at least 3 months. The initial haematological response is a reticulocytosis which peaks on the fifth to seventh day. The Hb concentration must be followed until it reaches the normal range, because a few patients, especially those with the malabsorption syndrome, may also be vitamin B_{12}- or iron-deficient; this can be detected by an incomplete rise in the Hb level. Such patients show a second response when vitamin B_{12} or iron is added to their treatment.

Disturbances in vitamin B$_{12}$ or folate metabolism

Nitrous oxide (N$_2$O) disturbs vitamin B$_{12}$ metabolism by oxidizing and inactivating methylcobalamin (Chanarin 1982). Continuous exposure of patients to a mixture of 50% N$_2$O and 50% O$_2$ for 5–24 hours often induces mild megaloblastic changes in the marrow. Intermittent exposure to N$_2$O for prolonged periods has caused a neuropathy in dentists working with, or addicted to, this gas. Drugs which inhibit dihydrofolate reductase (e.g. methotrexate and pyrimethamine) cause macrocytosis and megaloblastic changes by interfering with the regeneration of 5,10-methylenetetrahydrofolate from dihydrofolate. Megaloblastic haemopoiesis is also seen in some rare congenital disorders of vitamin B$_{12}$ and folate metabolism.

Vitamin B$_{12}$- and folate-independent causes of megaloblastic haemopoiesis

A list of conditions causing megaloblastic haemopoiesis by mechanisms unrelated to vitamin B$_{12}$ or folate is given in Table 5.4. The drugs listed interfere with nucleic acid synthesis. Orotic aciduria is a rare inherited disorder in which megaloblastic anaemia develops because of a reduced activity of enzymes involved in the conversion of orotic acid to uridine monophosphate. This leads to an impairment in the supply of pyrimidine bases for incorporation into DNA and RNA.

Table 5.4 Vitamin B$_{12}$-independent and folate-independent causes of macrocytosis with megaloblastic haemopoiesis.

OTHER CAUSES OF MEGALOBLASTS

Abnormalities of nucleic acid synthesis
Drug therapy
   Antipurines (mercaptopurine, azathioprine)
   Antipyrimidines (fluorouracil)
   Others (hydroxyurea)
Orotic aciduria

Uncertain aetiology
Myelodysplastic syndromes*, erythroleukaemia
Some congenital dyserythropoietic anaemias

* Some patients show normoblastic erythropoiesis.

MACROCYTOSIS WITH NORMOBLASTS

Normal neonates (physiological)
Chronic alcoholism*
Chronic liver disease*
Haemolytic anaemia
Hypothyroidism
Therapy with anticonvulsant drugs*
Normal pregnancy
Chronic lung disease (with hypoxia)
Myelodysplastic syndromes*
Hypoplastic and aplastic anaemia

* Some patients show B_{12}- and folate-independent
megaloblastic erythropoiesis.

Table 5.5 Causes of vitamin B_{12}- and folate-independent macrocytosis with normoblastic erythropoiesis.

Macrocytosis associated with normoblastic erythropoiesis

There are a number of conditions in which high MCVs may be associated with normoblastic erythropoiesis (Table 5.5). The most common of these, and indeed the commonest cause of macrocytosis in the UK, is chronic alcoholism.

CHRONIC ALCOHOLISM

With the advent of automated blood counting machines which estimate red-cell indices on every blood sample analysed, relatively accurate estimates of MCV have become available on a large number of patients. Such data have revealed that the prevalence of macrocytosis which is not due to B_{12} or folate deficiency, is higher than previously thought and that many individuals showing this abnormality consumed excess quantities of alcohol (Unger & Johnson 1974). It seems that the level of alcohol consumption that induces macrocytosis varies considerably in different individuals. Only about 35% of individuals who consume 100–800 g (mean 380 g) alcohol per day (i.e. an average of a bottle of spirits or its equivalent each day) develop MCVs above the normal range (Wickramasinghe et al. 1994). Although some chronic alcoholics suffer from folate deficiency due to inadequate intake, the majority have neither B_{12} or folate deficiency, nor anaemia. When folate stores are adequate, erythropoiesis is usually normoblastic, not megaloblastic. It has been suggested that the macrocytosis is due to a toxic effect of acetaldehyde on erythroblasts. The acetaldehyde is probably generated locally by oxidation of ethanol by bone marrow macrophages. MCV values return to normal 2–3 months after stopping the high alcohol intake.

HAEMOLYTIC ANAEMIA

Some patients with haemolytic anaemia develop increasing macrocytosis and megaloblastic haemopoiesis due to folate deficiency (p. 41). Other patients develop macrocytosis by a mechanism that is unrelated to folate deficiency. In the latter, the macrocytosis is associated with normoblastic erythropoiesis and is a manifestation of greatly accelerated erythropoiesis. The reticulocytes produced under these circumstances are larger than normal and mature into macrocytes which differ from those seen in vitamin B_{12} or folate deficiency in having rounded rather than oval outlines.

HYPOTHYROIDISM

There is a high frequency of thyroid and parietal cell antibodies in both hypothyroidism and pernicious anaemia and about 10% of all patients with hypothyroidism have pernicious anaemia. Patients with hypothyroidism may also develop macrocytosis by a mechanism which is based not on B_{12} or folate deficiency but on the deficiency of thyroxine. About one-quarter of patients with hypothyroidism (without associated pernicious anaemia) have an MCV above the normal range. Following the administration of thyroxine, all patients, including those whose MCV is within the normal range, show a fall in MCV (Horton et al. 1976).

ANTICONVULSANT DRUGS

A high MCV is seen in some patients receiving phenytoin sodium (with or without other anticonvulsant drugs) and this may be associated either with megaloblastic or normoblastic erythropoiesis. In a proportion of patients with megaloblastic changes, the macrocytosis is caused by folate deficiency and such patients are often anaemic. In the other patients with megaloblastic changes, and in all patients with normoblastic erythropoiesis, the macrocytosis is caused by an unknown mechanism independent of vitamin B_{12} and folate abnormalities; such patients are usually not anaemic.

References

Ardeman S., Chanarin I. (1965) Assay of gastric intrinsic factor in the diagnosis of Addisonian pernicious anaemia. Br. J. Haematol. **11**, 305–314.
Carmel R. (1990) Subtle and atypical cobalamin deficiency states. Am. J. Hematol. **34**, 108–114.
Chanarin I. (1982) The effects of nitrous oxide on cobalamins, folates and on related events. In: CRC Critical Reviews on Toxicology, pp. 179–213. CRC Press, Florida.

Chanarin I., Rothman D., Ward A., Perry J. (1968) Folate status and requirement in pregnancy. *Br. Med. J.* **21**, 390–394.

Chanarin I., Deacon R., Lumb M., Perry J. (1980) Vitamin B_{12} regulates folate metabolism by the supply of formate. *Lancet* **2**, 505–507.

Deller L.J., Witts L.J. (1962) Changes in the blood after partial gastrectomy with special reference to vitamin B_{12}. *Q. J. Med.* **31**, 71–88.

Giles C. (1966) An account of 335 cases of megaloblastic anaemia of pregnancy and the puerperium. *J. Clin. Pathol.* **19**, 1–11.

Glesson P.A., Toh B.H. (1991) Molecular targets in pernicious anaemia. *Immunol. Today* **12**, 233–238.

Healton E.H., Savage D.G., Brust J.C.M., Garrett T.J., Lindenbaum J. (1991) Neurologic aspects of cobalamin deficiency. *Medicine* **70**, 229–245.

Herbert V. (1964) Studies of folate deficiency in man. *Proc. R. Soc. Med.* **57**, 377–384.

Horton L., Coburn R.J., England J.M., Himsworth R.L. (1976) The haematology of hypothyroidism. *Q. J. Med.* **45**, 101–123.

Pant S.H., Ashbury A.K., Richardson E.P. (1968) The myelopathy of pernicious anaemia. A neuropathological reappraisal. *Acta Neurol. Scand.* **44**, Suppl. **35**, 1–36.

Schilling R.F. (1953) Intrinsic factor studies. II. The effect of gastric juice on the urinary excretion of radioactivity after the oral administration of radioactive vitamin B_{12}. *J. Lab. Clin. Med.* **42**, 860–866.

Stabler S.P., Allen R.H., Savage D.G., Lindenbaum J. (1990) Clinical spectrum and diagnosis of cobalamin deficiency. *Blood* **76**, 871–881.

Unger K.W., Johnson D., Jr. (1974) Red blood cell mean corpuscular volume: a potential indicator of alcohol usage in a working population. *Am. J. Med. Sci.* **267**, 281–289.

Wickramasinghe S.N. (1972) Kinetics and morphology of haemopoiesis in pernicious anaemia (Annotation). *Br. J. Haematol.* **22**, 111–115.

Wickramasinghe S.N., Corridan B., Hasan R., Marjot D.H. (1994) Correlations between acetaldehyde-modified haemoglobin, carbohydrate-deficient transferrin (CDT) and haematological abnormalities in chronic alcoholism. *Alcohol Alcohol.* **29**, 415–423.

Reviews

Bhatt H.R., James V.H.T., Besser G.M., Bottazzo G.F., Keen H. (1994) *Advances in Thomas Addison's Diseases*, Vols 1 & 2. Journal of Endocrinology Ltd, Bristol.

Chanarin I. (1990) *The Megaloblastic Anaemias*, 3rd edn. Blackwell Scientific Publications, Oxford.

Wickramasinghe S.N. (ed.) (1995) *Megaloblastic Anaemia*. In: Baillière's Clinical Haematology, International Practice and Research, Vol 8/No 3. Baillière Tindall, London.

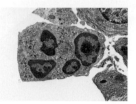

Conditions Causing White Cell Abnormalities

Objectives in learning

1 To know the more common conditions causing reductions and increases in the absolute counts of various types of white cell in the blood.

2 To be familiar with the aetiology, pathogenesis, clinical and haematological features and method of diagnosis of infectious mononucleosis.

3 To be aware of some of the inherited and acquired causes of abnormal granulocyte morphology and function.

In pathological states, circulating white blood cells may show alterations in their morphology, function or concentration. Although changes in the absolute count of various types of white cell are commonly found in disease and are usually non-specific, they may provide invaluable diagnostic clues. Alterations in white cells are most frequently associated with non-neoplastic disorders but may also be seen in the myelodysplastic syndromes (a pre-leukaemic state), in the chronic myeloproliferative disorders, and in various malignant diseases, including leukaemias.

Leucopenia

The terms 'leucopenia' and 'neutropenia' are used to describe a reduction in the total white cell count and neutrophil count, respectively, to values below their normal ranges. The terms 'lymphocytopenia' or 'lymphopenia' are used when the lymphocyte count is subnormal.

NEUTROPENIA

Selective neutropenia may occur in a large number of conditions (Table 6.1). In particular, it may be found in patients receiving various drugs, many of which are in common use. There is a substantial risk of serious infection when the neutrophil count falls below $0.5 \times 10^9/l$.

CAUSES OF SELECTIVE NEUTROPENIA

Physiological
Neutropenia in blacks (see p. 7)

Certain drugs
Anti-inflammatory drugs: indomethacin, oxyphenbutazone,
   phenylbutazone, sodium aurothiomalate
Anti-bacterial drugs: chloramphenicol, co-trimoxazole
   (sulphamethoxazole-trimethoprim), other sulphonamides
Some anticonvulsants, antidiabetic drugs, antithyroid drugs,
   antimalarial drugs, tranquillizers, antidepressants and antihistamines

Infections
Bacterial: overwhelming pyogenic infections, brucellosis, typhoid,
   miliary tuberculosis
Some viral, protozoal and fungal infections

Immune neutropenia
SLE, Felty's syndrome, autoimmune neutropenia, neonatal alloimmune
   neutropenia, aminopyrine-induced agranulocytosis

Miscellaneous
Hypothyroidism, hypopituitarism, cyclical neutropenia, familial benign
   chronic neutropenia

Table 6.1

Neutropenia is also found as part of pancytopenia; the main causes of pancytopenia are given in Table 9.3 on p. 180.

Agranulocytosis

The term 'agranulocytosis' was originally used to refer to an acute febrile illness with necrotizing lesions of the mouth and throat associated with an extreme reduction or complete absence of neutrophil granulocytes in the peripheral blood. It is a rare condition and is now known to be caused by severe drug-induced neutropenia. The platelets and red cells are not affected. The first drug to be incriminated was aminopyrine, and although this compound is no longer prescribed, it is still available in some proprietary preparations in certain parts of the world. Many other drugs will occasionally cause agranulocytosis. These include: some antithyroid drugs, especially thiouracil; certain tranquillizers such as chlorpromazine; some antibacterial drugs such as sulphonamides and chloramphenicol; and several anti-inflammatory drugs, including phenylbutazone and gold salts. Many of these drugs may also cause aplastic anaemia. The mechanism of action of these drugs, when known, is either through an antigen–antibody reaction or through interference with one or more metabolic processes in neutrophil precursors (e.g. suppression of DNA synthesis by chlorpromazine).

Agranulocytosis should always be considered in a patient presenting with a severe infection of the throat and sometimes elsewhere, accompanied by profound weakness and exhaustion. The treatment is withdrawal of any suspected drug and use of appropriate antibiotics. The mortality rate is high; the prognosis is better if there are some white-cell precursors in the marrow than when these are absent.

LYMPHOCYTOPENIA (LYMPHOPENIA)

Lymphocytopenia is seen after the administration of corticosteroids, following trauma or surgery, in many acute infections or after high-dose radiotherapy or therapy with cytotoxic drugs. It is also found in Cushing's syndrome, uraemia, systemic lupus erythematosus (SLE), sarcoidosis, Hodgkin's disease and in certain immunodeficiency syndromes, including AIDS.

Leucocytosis

An increase in the absolute count of white blood cells, neutrophils, eosinophils, basophils, monocytes and lymphocytes above the normal range is described, respectively, as leucocytosis, neutrophil leucocytosis, eosinophil leucocytosis (eosinophilia), basophil leucocytosis, monocytosis and lymphocytosis.

NEUTROPHIL LEUCOCYTOSIS

This is the most common abnormality of white blood cells. The causes of neutrophil leucocytosis are many (Peterson & Hrisinko 1993) and are summarized in Table 6.2. An important cause is infection by pyogenic organisms. Here, the neutrophil counts are usually in the range 10 to $30 \times 10^9/l$, but may be higher. In addition, there may be increased numbers of neutrophil band cells, some neutrophil metamyelocytes and myelocytes, and very occasional myeloblasts on the blood film ('shift to the left' or 'left shift'). The neutrophils may also show toxic granulation or Döhle bodies or both, and the neutrophil alkaline phosphatase score is raised (see p. 131). Toxic granules are abnormally coarse, reddish-violet (azurophilic) granules which are diffusely distributed throughout the cytoplasm; Döhle bodies are 1–2 μm long, pale greyish-blue cytoplas-

CAUSES OF NEUTROPHIL LEUCOCYTOSIS

Physiological
Neonates, exercise, emotion, pregnancy, parturition, lactation

Pathological
Acute infections: especially by pyogenic bacteria
Acute inflammation not caused by infections: surgery, burns, infarcts, crush injuries, rheumatoid arthritis, myositis, vasculitis
Acute haemorrhage and acute haemolysis
Metabolic: uraemia, diabetic ketoacidosis, gout, acute thyrotoxicosis
Non-haematological malignancies: carcinoma, lymphoma, melanoma
Chronic myeloproliferative disorders: chronic granulocytic leukaemia, polycythaemia rubra vera, myelofibrosis
Drugs: adrenaline, corticosteroids, G-CSF and GM-CSF (p. 20)
Miscellaneous: convulsions, paroxysmal tachycardia, electric shock, post-neutropenic rebound neutrophilia, post-splenectomy

Table 6.2

mic inclusions, which are usually situated at the periphery of the cell (Romanowsky stain). A 'shift to the left', toxic granulation and Döhle bodies reflect accelerated neutrophil granulocytopoiesis and may be seen not only in acute infections but also in non-infective inflammatory states (e.g. severe burns), in normal pregnancy and in patients with various malignant neoplasms.

Whereas adults respond to acute bacterial infections with a neutrophil leucocytosis, young children may respond with a lymphocytosis.

The neutrophil leucocytosis seen after exercise, in emotional states, after the administration of adrenaline, after electric shocks and in patients with convulsions and paroxysmal tachycardia are caused by a rapid shift of neutrophils from the marginated to the circulating granulocyte pool (p. 7).

EOSINOPHIL LEUCOCYTOSIS (EOSINOPHILIA)

Eosinophilia is usually caused by allergic disorders or parasitic infestations. The parasites that provoke the highest eosinophil counts are metazoa which invade tissues. Some causes of eosinophilia are given in Table 6.3 (Beeson & Bass 1977; Mahmoud et al. 1980).

Idiopathic hypereosinophilic syndrome

Very high eosinophil counts, sometimes accompanied by anaemia and

CAUSES OF EOSINOPHILIA

Parasitic infestations: filariasis, hookworm, ascariasis, strongyloidiasis, schistosomiasis, toxocariasis, trichinosis, hydatid cyst, scabies

Allergic disorders: bronchial asthma, hay fever, allergic vasculitis, Stevens–Johnson syndrome, drug sensitivity (e.g. chlorpromazine, penicillin, sulphonamides)

Recovery from acute infection

Skin diseases: eczema, psoriasis, pemphigus, dermatitis herpetiformis

Pulmonary eosinophilia: Loeffler's syndrome (pulmonary infiltration with eosinophilia)

Polyarteritis nodosa

Chronic granulocytic leukaemia, eosinophilic leukaemia (rare)

Other malignant diseases: Hodgkin's disease, angioimmunoblastic lymphadenopathy, carcinoma (usually with metastases)

Idiopathic hypereosinophilic syndrome

Table 6.3

thrombocytopenia are found in a disorder of uncertain aetiology named the idiopathic hypereosinophilic syndrome (*Lancet* 1983; Liesveld & Abboud 1992). The clinical features of this disorder include fever, night sweats, weight loss, splenomegaly, damage to the heart, lungs and nervous system and thromboembolic episodes.

Cardiac damage is a characteristic feature. Lesions consist of areas of eosinophilic infiltration, muscle necrosis and fibrosis mainly affecting the endocardium and subendocardial myocardium; they have been attributed to the cytotoxic effects of a constituent of eosinophil granules. Patients may be treated with prednisone, hydroxyurea or both. In some cases, the idiopathic hypereosinophilic syndrome appears to be primarily a disease of the bone marrow and terminates in acute leukaemia.

BASOPHIL LEUCOCYTOSIS (BASOPHILIA)
The causes of basophilia include hypersensitivity reactions, myxoedema and chronic myeloproliferative disorders.

MONOCYTOSIS
A high monocyte count ($>0.8 \times 10^9/l$) is characteristic of certain bacterial infections, notably brucellosis, tuberculosis, typhoid fever and

CAUSES OF MONOCYTOSIS

Bacterial infections: tuberculosis, brucellosis, syphilis, subacute bacterial endocarditis, typhoid, recovery from acute infections

Protozoal infections: leishmaniasis, malaria, trypanosomiasis

Rickettsial infections: typhus, Rocky Mountain spotted fever

Myelodysplastic syndromes

Leukaemias: monocytic and myelomonocytic leukaemias, chronic granulocytic leukaemia

Other malignant diseases: Hodgkin's disease, carcinoma, malignant histiocytosis

Miscellaneous: ulcerative colitis, Crohn's disease

Table 6.4

CAUSES OF LYMPHOCYTOSIS

Viral infections: infectious mononucleosis (glandular fever), cytomegalovirus infection, rubella, chicken pox, measles, mumps, influenza, infectious hepatitis

Bacterial infections: pertussis, other acute bacterial infections in infants and young children, tuberculosis, brucellosis, syphilis.

Chronic lymphocytic leukaemia

Lymphomas and Waldenström's macroglobulinaemia

Post-splenectomy (often temporary)

Table 6.5

subacute bacterial endocarditis. Other conditions associated with a monocytosis (Maldonado & Hanlon 1965) are given in Table 6.4.

LYMPHOCYTOSIS

Lymphocytosis ($>3.5 \times 10^9$ lymphocytes/l in adults) is the usual response to many viral infections. In infectious mononucleosis (see p. 129), the high lymphocyte count is associated with the presence of large, atypical mononuclear cells (which are activated T-lymphocytes). The one acute bacterial infection which is characteristically accompanied by very high lymphocyte counts, sometimes in excess of 50×10^9/l, is whooping cough (pertussis). Many other acute bacterial infections, which cause neutrophil leucocytosis in adults, may provoke a lymphocytosis in infants and young children. The various causes of lymphocytosis (Peterson & Hrisinko 1993) are listed in Table 6.5.

Infectious mononucleosis (glandular fever)

This is a usually benign infectious disease in which the epithelial cells of the nasopharynx and B-lymphocytes are infected by the Epstein–Barr virus (EBV) (Banatvala 1970; Pullen 1973; Chetham & Roberts 1991; Straus et al. 1993). EBV is a DNA virus belonging to the herpesvirus group. The virus is found in the saliva intermittently for 12–18 months after recovery from glandular fever; transmission is by droplets or by kissing. The incubation period is about 5–7 weeks. A high proportion of individuals become infected early in childhood and over 90% of adults have EBV-related antibodies. Most of those infected have subclinical or mild attacks; this is particularly true of children. The syndrome of glandular fever is usually seen in adolescents and young adults. The most common symptoms are malaise and fatigue, sweats, sore throat and dysphagia, anorexia, nausea, headaches and fever. Pharyngitis and follicular tonsillitis are often seen. In most cases, there is bilateral cervical lymphadenopathy and in some cases there may also be enlargement of axillary and inguinal glands. In about half the patients, there is mild or moderate splenomegaly and in about 20%, there is slight hepatomegaly. Some patients have periorbital oedema and a small number have a maculopapular skin rash or jaundice. Very occasionally, there may be life-threatening splenic rupture. Other infrequent complications are thrombocytopenic purpura, autoimmune haemolytic anaemia (cold antibody with anti-i or, less often, anti-I specificity), aplastic anaemia, severe hepatitis, ECG abnormalities, pericarditis, myocarditis, pulmonary involvement or nervous system involvement. The latter includes encephalitis, meningitis, Guillain–Barré syndrome, optic neuritis, cranial nerve palsies and myelitis (Connelly & De Witt 1994).

Diagnosis

The two characteristic findings in the peripheral blood are, an increase in the absolute lymphocyte count above the normal upper limit of $3.5 \times 10^9/l$, usually up to $10–20 \times 10^9/l$, and the appearance of lymphocytes with abnormal morphology, often described as atypical mononuclear cells or atypical lymphocytes (Fig. 6.1, Plates 4, 5). The atypical mononuclear cells appear after the first week of the illness and may persist for up to 1 or 2 months. The morphology of these cells is variable and very similar to that of peripheral blood lymphocytes which have transformed following stimulation with mitogens in vitro. The abnormal

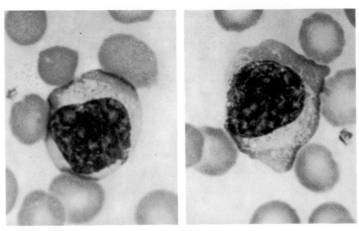

Fig. 6.1 Two atypical mononuclear cells from the blood film of a patient with glandular fever. As is commonly the case, the cytoplasmic basophilia is more marked at the periphery of the cell. Both cells are larger than normal lymphocytes.

cells are large, have moderately abundant very basophilic cytoplasm, possess a lobulated or indented nucleus with a relatively fine chromatin pattern and prominent nucleoli, and display a scalloped margin at points of contact with other cells on a blood film (Carter 1966). The atypical mononuclear cells are cytotoxic and suppressor T-lymphocytes; the cytotoxic T cells are reacting against infected B-lymphocytes which have virus-encoded antigens on their surface (only B-cells have a receptor for EBV). Most of the infected B cells are morphologically normal and the absolute B-lymphocyte count is increased. Atypical mononuclear cells are not diagnostic of infectious mononucleosis, being also found in other viral infections (e.g. cytomegalovirus (CMV), hepatitis A or adenovirus infection and acute HIV infection), following immunization, and in hypersensitivity reactions to drugs.

In most patients with glandular fever, heterophile antibodies develop. These are antibodies formed in response to antigens of one species, which cross-react with antigens on the cells of other species. The most characteristic heterophile antibody agglutinates sheep and horse red cells and is absorbed by ox red cells but not by guinea pig kidney. The Paul–Bunnell test and other simpler tests for glandular fever (e.g. the monospot test) are based on the detection of this antibody which develops in 80–90% of patients during the second and third weeks of the illness; the antibody declines and is usually undetectable after 2–3 months. IgG antibodies aganist viral capsid antigen (VCA) also appear at the same time and persist for years, giving lasting immunity. The presence of IgM antibody to VCA is diagnostic of a recent or continuing infection. Antibodies to the Epstein–Barr nuclear antigens (EBNA) appear about 1 month after the onset of the illness and persist throughout life.

Leukaemoid reactions

Occasionally, patients are seen in whom the peripheral blood findings suggest at first sight that they could have leukaemia, but in reality the changes are an unusual response to some other disorder. The total white cell count is over $50 \times 10^9/l$ and the blood picture may resemble that seen in chronic granulocytic leukaemia (CGL) or chronic lymphocytic leukaemia. Leukaemoid reactions resembling acute leukaemia are rare but may be found in disseminated tuberculosis and in Down's syndrome (during the neonatal period).

In the type simulating CGL, there are many immature white cells (myelocytes, promyelocytes and a few myeloblasts) in the peripheral blood. This abnormal reaction sometimes occurs as the result of severe infection, especially in children, and also in patients with malignant tumours, rapid haemolysis and burns. The following characteristics of granulocytic leukaemoid reactions help to distinguish them from chronic granulocytic leukaemia: the neutrophils may show toxic granulation and Döhle bodies (Plates 23, 24), the basophil and eosinophil counts are not raised, and the alkaline phosphatase score in the polymorphs is normal or increased, not reduced as in CGL.

Lymphocytic leukaemoid reactions may be seen as an 'excessive' response to infection, usually in infectious mononucleosis and pertussis.

Leucoerythroblastic reaction

The characteristic feature is the presence of a number of nucleated red cells (erythroblasts) as well as immature white cells (mainly myelocytes) in the peripheral blood film. The total white-cell count may or may not be elevated. A leucoerythroblastic blood picture may be found when the bone marrow is infiltrated with malignant cells (carcinoma (Plate 40), lymphoma, myeloma, leukaemia), fibrous tissue (primary or secondary myelofibrosis) or storage cells (e.g. Gaucher's disease). It may also occur after severe haemorrhage and when there is marked haemolysis. A bone marrow aspiration and a trephine biopsy of the marrow often help to establish the diagnosis.

INHERITED NEUTROPHIL ABNORMALITIES

Condition	Inheritance, prevalence	Characteristics
Pelger–Huet anomaly	Autosomal dominant 1:1000–10 000	Heterozygotes have bilobed spectacle-like neutrophil nuclei, homozygotes have round or oval neutrophil nuclei, asymptomatic
Neutrophil myeloperoxidase deficiency	Autosomal recessive 1:2000	Detected during automated differential counting based on cytochemistry, usually asymptomatic
Chediak–Higashi syndrome	Autosomal recessive	Giant granules in leucocytes, neutropenia, thrombocytopenia, partial albinism, hepato-splenomegaly, death in infancy or early childhood from infection and haemorrhage
Chronic granulomatous disease	Majority X-linked, some autosomal recessive	Normal neutrophil morphology, inability to kill ingested microorganisms due to absence of cytochrome b_{558} or other components of the respiratory burst oxidase (p. 11) leading to impaired superoxide generation, recurrent granulomatous lesions from early childhood

Table 6.6 Some inherited abnormalities of neutrophil morphology or function or both.

Abnormalities of granulocyte morphology and function

There are a number of inherited conditions causing abnormalities in granulocyte morphology or function or both. The essential features of some of these are summarized in Table 6.6. The most common acquired abnormalities of neutrophil morphology include 'shift to the left' (p.125), hypersegmentation of the nucleus (p. 99), toxic granulation (p. 125), Döhle bodies (p. 125), hypogranularity (p. 175) and the acquired Pelger–Huet anomaly (p. 175). Acquired abnormalities of neutrophil function, such as impaired chemotactic mobility, phagocytosis or killing, have been reported in a large number of conditions including corticosteroid therapy, hypophosphataemia, alcoholism, acute or chronic myeloid leukaemia, myelodysplasia and the chronic myeloproliferative disorders.

References

Banatvala J.E. (1970) Infectious mononucleosis. Recent developments. (Annotation.) *Br. J. Haematol.* **19**, 129–133.

Beeson P.B., Bass D.A. (1977) *The Eosinophil.* W.B. Saunders, Philadelphia.

Carter R.L. (1966) Review of some recent observations on 'glandular fever cells'. *J. Clin. Pathol.* **19**, 448–455.

Chetham M.M., Roberts K.B. (1991) Infectious mononucleosis in adolescents. *Pediatr. Ann.* **20**, 206–213.

Connelly K.P., De Witt L.D. (1994) Neurologic complications of infectious mononucleosis. *Pediatr. Neurol.* **10**, 181–184.

Lancet (Editorial) (1983) The hypereosinophilic syndrome. *Lancet* **i**, 1417.

Liesveld J.L., Abboud C.N. (1992) Hypereosinophilic syndromes: an update. *Int. J. Clin. Lab. Res.* **22**, 5–10.

Mahmoud A.A.F., Austen K.F., Simon A.S. (1980) *The Eosinophil in Health and Disease.* Grune & Stratton, New York.

Maldonado J.E., Hanlon D.G. (1965) Monocytosis: a current appraisal. *Mayo Clin. Proc.* **40**, 248–259.

Peterson L., Hrisinko M.A. (1993) Benign lymphocytosis and reactive neutrophilia. Laboratory features provide diagnostic clues. *Clin. Lab. Med.* **13**, 863–877.

Pullen H. (1973) Infectious mononucleosis. *Br. Med. J.* **2**, 350–352.

Straus S.E., Cohen J.I., Tosato G., Meier J. (1993) Epstein–Barr virus infections: biology, pathogenesis and management. *Ann. Intern. Med.* **118**, 45–58.

CHAPTER 7

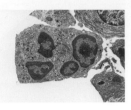

Acute and
Chronic Leukaemias

Objectives in learning

1 To understand the classification of leukaemia into acute lympho-blastic, acute myeloid, chronic lymphocytic and chronic granulocytic based on the clinical picture and the cytological findings, and to be aware of further schemes for subclassifying the acute leukaemias.

2 To have a broad understanding of the nature of leukaemia and of aetiological factors in haematological neoplasia; to understand pathogenetic mechanisms responsible for clinical and laboratory features of these diseases.

3 To know the natural history of the main types of leukaemia and the effects of treatment on it.

4 To know the basic principles (but not the details) of treatment in: (a) acute leukaemia; (b) chronic granulocytic leukaemia; and (c) chronic lymphocytic leukaemia.

General considerations

The leukaemias are neoplasms of the precursors of blood cells and are characterized by the accumulation of abnormal white cells in the bone marrow; the neoplastic cells usually circulate in the blood and infiltrate tissues. Leukaemias are clonal disorders; that is, they arise from the neoplastic transformation usually of a single cell. In about 20% of cases of acute leukaemia and in chronic granulocytic leukaemia, the cell undergo-ing the transformation is probably a pluripotent stem cell (i.e. the cell which eventually gives rise to all types of blood cell, including lymphocytes). In other cases, the leukaemia seems to arise from a more mature progenitor cell which may be restricted to only one to three lines of differentiation. By repeated cell division, the transformed cell gener-ates an expanding clone of neoplastic cells. In acute leukaemias the neoplastic clone is of high malignancy and in chronic leukaemias it is of low malignancy. Leukaemic cells fail to mature or mature abnormally (acute leukaemias) or mature into cells with more or less normal mor-phology (chronic leukaemias).

Classification

There are four common varieties of leukaemia: acute lymphoblastic, acute myeloid, chronic lymphocytic and chronic granulocytic (chronic myeloid). The terms 'acute' and 'chronic' refer to the clinical course in untreated patients; those with acute leukaemia usually die within weeks or months and those with chronic leukaemias usually survive longer. This clinical subdivision of leukaemia corresponds with the degree of maturity of the predominant leukaemic cell type found in the bone marrow and blood, in that immature, blast-like cells predominate in many acute leukaemias and more mature cells predominate in chronic leukaemias. The predominant cell types found in the four common types of leukaemia are shown in Table 7.1. In the last decade, monoclonal antibodies against various cellular antigens and cytochemical techniques have been increasingly applied to characterize the leukaemic cells more finely and thus further to subdivide the acute leukaemias. One currently popular classification is based on the proposals of a French-American-British (FAB) cooperative group (Bennett et al. 1976; Bennett et al. 1980). The details of such classifications of the acute leukaemias are given in Tables 7.2–7.4 in order to illustrate the heterogeneity in the cytology of the leukaemic cell clone found both in acute lymphoblastic and in acute myeloid leukaemia.

PREDOMINANT ABNORMAL CELL TYPES

Type of leukaemia	Predominant leukaemic cell type in bone marrow and blood
Acute lymphoblastic	Lymphoblasts
Acute myeloid	Usually myeloblasts. Sometimes promyelocytes, monoblasts or promonocytes. Occasionally erythroblasts and, rarely, megakaryoblasts
Chronic lymphocytic	Lymphocytes
Chronic granulocytic (chronic myeloid)	Neutrophil myelocytes and metamyelocytes, and neutrophil granulocytes

Table 7.1 Predominant abnormal cell types in the major forms of leukaemia.

ACUTE LYMPHOBLASTIC LEUKAEMIA

FAB category	Features of leukaemic lymphoblasts
L1	Small; scanty cytoplasm; uniform appearance
L2	Large; more cytoplasm; heterogeneous in size and shape
L3	Large; moderately abundant basophilic cytoplasm; cytoplasmic vacuolation; cells are similar to those in Burkitt's lymphoma

*Beyond the core requirements of medical students but helps the understanding of general concepts.

Table 7.2* FAB classification of acute lymphoblastic leukaemia (L1–L3) (Bennett *et al.* 1976).

ACUTE MYELOID LEUKAEMIA

FAB category	Features of the bone marrow
M1, myeloblastic leukaemia without maturation	Myeloblasts predominate, most show little or no maturation
M2, myeloblastic leukaemia with maturation	Myeloblasts predominate, some show maturation to and beyond promyelocyte stage
M3, promyelocytic leukaemia	Promyelocytes predominate and are often hypergranular
M4, myelomonocytic leukaemia	Evidence of both granulocytic and monocytic maturation; promonocytes plus monocytes >20% in blood or marrow
M5, monocytic leukaemia	Monoblasts or promonocytes predominate
M6, erythroleukaemia	Presence of a high proportion of erythroblasts, often with marked morphological abnormalities
M7, megakaryoblastic leukaemia	Megakaryoblasts or micromegakaryocytes prominent. May be associated with acute myelofibrosis

*Beyond the core requirements of medical students but helps the understanding of general concepts.

Table 7.3* FAB classification of acute myeloid leukaemia (M1–M7) (Bennett *et al.* 1976, 1980).

IMMUNOLOGICAL CLASSIFICATION OF ALL

Category	Percentage cases of childhood ALL	Phenotype of leukaemic cells/presumed cell of origin	Corresponding FAB category
T-ALL	15–20	Thymocytes	L1 and L2
Pre-B-ALL	20	Pre-B-cells (have cytoplasmic μ-chains)	L1 and L2
B-ALL	1–2	Mature B cells (have surface membrane Ig)	L3 and L2
Common-ALL	50	Non-T, non-B-ALL. c-ALL antigen positive. Corresponds to an early cell committed to the B-cell lineage	L1 and L2
Null-ALL	8	Non-T, non-B-ALL. c-ALL antigen negative. Probably more immature than cells in c-ALL	L1 and L2

*Beyond the core requirements of medical students but helps the understanding of general concepts.

Table 7.4* Classification of acute lymphoblastic leukaemias (ALL) based on immunological markers.

Aetiology of leukaemia

The aetiology of leukaemia is still under investigation. Studies with inbred strains of mice have shown that the susceptibility of a mouse to develop leukaemia is based on a complex interaction between its genetic make-up and other factors such as its age, hormonal and immunological status and the degree of exposure to radiation or to leukaemogenic chemicals or viruses. For example, some strains of mice (e.g. C3H) rarely develop leukaemia spontaneously even in old age but readily do so after X-irradiation. By contrast, other strains (e.g. Ak) regularly develop leukaemia in old age. The development of leukaemia in humans also seems to depend on an interplay between multiple factors. Furthermore, leukaemogenesis seems to occur by a process involving multiple steps. The factors thought to be involved in human leukaemogenesis and the evidence in support of their involvement are discussed below.

IONIZING RADIATION

The evidence that ionizing radiation is leukaemogenic in humans is very good and is based on finding an increased incidence of leukaemia in:

1 the survivors of nuclear bomb explosions at Hiroshima and Nagasaki (i.e. individuals receiving a single large dose of whole-body ionizing radiation), and

2 patients with ankylosing spondylitis who had received repeated irradiation to the spine.

Several features of leukaemia that follow whole or partial body irradiation are worthy of note. These are:

1 there is a direct correlation between the dose of irradiation received and the risk of developing leukaemia;

2 only a proportion of heavily irradiated individuals develop leukaemia (e.g. only 1 per 60 of the heavily irradiated atomic bomb victims developed leukaemia over 12 years);

3 there is often a substantial latent period (the peak incidence occurs 5 years after exposure), and

4 radiation induces acute and chronic myeloid leukaemia and acute lymphoblastic leukaemia but not chronic lymphocytic leukaemia.

The validity of the observation that there is an increased incidence of leukaemia in children born to mothers who have been submitted to diagnostic radiology during pregnancy has not yet been settled.

CHEMICALS

There is good evidence that benzene is both myelotoxic and leukaemogenic; myelosuppression usually precedes the emergence of leukaemia. There is also some epidemiological evidence implicating cigarette smoking in the aetiology of leukaemia. Treatment with alkylating agents (e.g. melphalan, thio-TEPA, chlorambucil, cyclophosphamide and nitrosoureas such as BCNU and CCNU) is associated with an increased risk of developing leukaemia, as is treatment with epipodophyllotoxins and procarbazine. In the case of melphalan, chlorambucil and cyclophosphamide this increased risk is seen even in patients treated for nonmalignant disorders.

VIRUSES

Viruses are involved in leukaemogenesis in mice, rats, chickens and cats. However, the main virus that has been implicated in human leukaemogenesis to date is the retrovirus human T-cell leukaemia virus I (HTLV-I), which can be isolated from patients with adult T-cell leukaemia/lymphoma (p. 200). This rare type of leukaemia/lymphoma is endemic in a localized area in Japan, but clusters and isolated cases have been found elsewhere, mainly in blacks in the West Indies and the USA. HTLV-I does not carry an oncogene and does not selectively integrate near a proto-oncogene. It produces a *trans*-acting regulatory molecule which affects the activity of cellular genes.

GENETIC FACTORS

Some of the evidence implicating genetic factors in human leukaemogenesis is not as straightforward as the evidence obtained from experiments on genetically pure strains of mice. For instance, it has been shown that following the development of acute leukaemia in one of a pair of identical twins, there is a 25% chance of the co-twin also doing so within weeks or months. Furthermore, there are a relatively small number of reports in which between two and four cases of leukaemia occurred in one or more generations of the same family. On first glance, these data may appear to indicate the operation of genetic factors. However, there is controversy as to whether the frequency with which two or more cases of leukaemia have been observed in the same family is greater than that which would be expected by chance. Furthermore, as families share a common environment, the data on leukaemia in twins and familial leukaemia do not necessarily indicate the operation of genetic factors in leukaemogenesis; they may equally indicate the operation of environmental factors. More definite evidence of the importance of genetic factors in human leukaemogenesis comes from a high incidence of acute myeloid leukaemia in patients with Down's syndrome (trisomy 21) and in the inherited genetic instability syndromes Fanconi's anaemia and Bloom's syndrome which are associated with multiple chromosomal breaks. Various acquired chromosomal abnormalities are seen in leukaemias (e.g. the Philadelphia (Ph) chromosome in chronic myeloid leukaemia) and the relevance of some of these, and of oncogenes, in leukaemogenesis is discussed below.

Oncogenes

The growth of normal cells is under the control of a number of cellular genes known as proto-oncogenes. The products of such genes and the ways in which they regulate normal cell proliferation have not yet been fully elucidated. Some proto-oncogenes seem to code for growth factors or transmembrane growth factor receptors. Others code for proteins involved in the transduction of signals from growth factor receptors at the cell surface to intracytoplasmic and intranuclear biochemical reactions regulating cell proliferation. There is evidence that in malignant cells, one or other of a number of genetic alterations affect proto-oncogenes which activate them into oncogenes (i.e. genes implicated in the generation of malignant change). In theory, activation of proto-oncogenes may be involved both in tumour initiation and in tumour progression (i.e. the evolution of the mutant clone, including the acquisition of malignant characteristics). The alterations known to activate proto-oncogenes include point mutations, insertion of viral genomes exerting transcriptional control near them, gene amplification (i.e. the generation of multiple gene copies) resulting in overexpression, and translocation into an actively transcribed locus.

Activation of certain proto-oncogenes has been reported in some human leukaemias and lymphomas (Cline 1994). For example, the formation of the Ph chromosome in virtually all cases of chronic granulocytic leukaemia and in 5–25% of cases of acute lymphoblastic leukaemia is associated with the activation of the *abl* proto-oncogene. The Ph chromosome is an abnormally small chromosome 22 formed by the reciprocal translocation of parts of the long arm of chromosomes 22 and 9 and this change is designated t(9;22) or, more precisely, t(9q+;22q−). The break point on chromosome 22 (situated in a breakpoint cluster region, BCR) is joined to the 3′ end of the *abl* proto-oncogene on chromosome 9 and this results in a BCR-*abl* fusion gene and the consequent synthesis of a BCR-*abl* fusion protein. The gene product of the *abl* gene is a cytoplasmic tyrosine kinase which catalyses the phosphorylation of tyrosine; this phosphorylation seems to influence cell growth. The BCR-*abl* fusion protein formed in chronic myeloid leukaemia has increased tyrosine kinase activity. Examples of oncogene activation in human leukaemias are given in Table 7.5. Interestingly, point mutations in the *ras* proto-oncogenes have been reported not only in the acute leukaemias but also, in 20–40% of patients with the pre-leukaemic conditions known as the myelodysplastic syndromes (p. 174) and, in 20% of patients with myeloma. Proto-oncogene activation also occurs in Burkitt's lymphoma; this is a high-grade B-cell lymphoma, not a leukaemia (p. 199). Here, translocation events juxtapose the *myc* proto-oncogene on chromosome 8 next to the heavy chain locus on chromosome 14 [t(8;14)] or, less frequently, the ϰ light chain locus on chromosome 2 [t(2;8)] or the λ light chain locus on chromosome 22 [t(8;22)]. The same translocation events occur in some cases of B-cell acute lymphoblastic leukaemia. In 85% of cases of follicular lymphoma and in some cases of diffuse lymphoma and B-chronic lymphocytic leukaemia, the t(14;18) translocation brings the *bcl*-2 proto-oncogene on chromosome 18 next to the heavy chain locus on chromosome 14 in such a way that despite activation of the fusion gene, there is a failure to synthesize any fusion protein; the *bcl*-2 protein is normally found in mitochondria and prevents the programmed death (apoptosis) of B cells.

ONCOGENES IN HUMAN LEUKAEMIAS

Disease	Proto-oncogene	Proto-oncogene protein	Event activating proto-oncogene	Prevalence of activation (%)	Effects of activation on cell function
CGL	abl	Cytoplasmic tyrosine kinase	t(9;22), BCR on chromosome 22 translocated into abl on chromosome 9	100	BCR-abl fusion protein (210 kD) with increased tyrosine kinase activity
Non T-ALL	abl	Cytoplasmic tyrosine kinase	t(9;22), BCR breakpoint differs from above	5–25	BCR-abl fusion protein (190 kD) with increased tyrosine kinase activity
Non T-ALL	N-ras	GTP-binding proteins involved in signal transduction	Point mutation	15	Mutant N-ras protein leading to altered intracellular signalling
AML	N-ras K-ras H-ras	GTP-binding proteins involved in signal transduction	Point mutation	25	Mutant ras protein leading to altered intracellular signalling
T-ALL	myc	Located in nucleus, function uncertain	t(8;14), myc on chromosome 8 translocated to T-cell receptor gene on chromosome 14	10–20	myc gene expression deregulated

CGL, chronic granulocytic leukaemia; ALL, acute lymphoblastic leukaemia; AML, acute myeloid leukaemia; t, chromosomal translocation; BCR, breakpoint cluster region on chromosome 22, including breakpoints involved in formation of Philadelphia chromosome.

Table 7.5 Some oncogenes involved in human leukaemias.

Recent studies have shown that in acute promyelocytic leukaemia (FAB category M3, Table 7.3) a 15;17 translocation results in the fusion of the retinoic acid receptor (RARα) gene locus on chromosome 17 with the promyelocytic leukaemia (PML) locus on chromosome 15. The abnormal retinoic acid receptor formed from the chimeric gene appears to be insensitive to normal concentrations of retinoic acid since its presence results in a failure of the normal differentiation of promyelocytes to granulocytes. Interestingly, this leukaemia responds to high doses of *trans*-retinoic acid which overcomes the block in the differentiation of promyelocytes.

It is possible that both chemical leukaemogens and leukaemogenic viruses can activate proto-oncogenes.

Tumour suppressor genes

The products of tumour suppressor genes (anti-oncogenes) inhibit cell proliferation or promote apoptosis (programmed cell death). Inactivation of two such genes, p53 and retinoblastoma 1 (Rb1), by mutation or deletion appears to be sometimes involved in the evolution of certain types of leukaemia and lymphoma to a more aggressive state (Cline 1994). These types are chronic granulocytic leukaemia, chronic lymphocytic leukaemia, Burkitt's lymphoma and adult T-cell leukaemia/lymphoma. A single copy of a suppressor gene may be adequate for tumour suppression activity, and an inherited loss of a tumour suppressor gene together with an acquired defect in the second copy underlies the susceptibility to some familial tumours (e.g. retinoblastoma).

Features common to all leukaemias

There are a number of features that are found in all the leukaemias. These are:

1   infiltration and replacement of normal bone marrow with leukaemic cells which causes anaemia, neutropenia and thrombocytopenia;

2   infiltration of other tissues and organs with leukaemic cells, and

3   an increase in the basal metabolic rate when the tumour mass is large, leading to excessive sweating and loss of weight.

The most common clinical manifestations of leukaemia are related to the bone marrow infiltration. Thus, anaemia causes lassitude, weakness and shortness of breath and the neutropenia, which is aggravated by cytotoxic therapy, causes bacterial infections (pneumonia and septicaemia). The thrombocytopenia leads to abnormal bleeding.

Gram-negative infections predominate, the patient's own intestinal flora often being the source of septicaemias. The organisms are usually *Escherichia coli*, *Klebsiella* or *Pseudomonas aeruginosa*. Gram-positive infections (e.g. with *Staphylococcus aureus*) also occur, and infections with unusual skin organisms such as *Staphylococcus epidermidis* may be seen consequent to the use of long term indwelling catheters. When cytotoxic therapy causes marked immunosuppression, opportunistic infections (i.e. infections rarely seen in immunologically normal individuals) may occur with organisms such as *Candida*, *Aspergillus* and *Pneumocystis carinii*. Immunosuppression may also be associated with generalized and fulminant infections with viruses such as herpes simplex and herpes zoster.

The haemorrhagic manifestations often consist of petechiae, epistaxis, bleeding from the gums and spontaneous bruising. Less commonly, bleeding may occur into other organs such as the nervous system, eye and internal ear.

The extent and nature of extramedullary tissue infiltration varies with both the type of leukaemia and the stage of progression of the disease. For example, whereas infiltration of lymph nodes is a common feature of the late stages of chronic lymphocytic leukaemia, it is unusual in acute myeloid leukaemia.

The acute leukaemias

Both acute lymphoblastic leukaemia (ALL) and acute myeloid leukaemia (AML) (Cartwright & Staines 1992) occur at all ages. However, ALL is the most common type of acute leukaemia in children and AML is the most common type in adults. The incidence of ALL is 1–2 per 100 000 population per year; the age distribution shows a distinct peak at 3–4 years. The incidence of AML is low in children and rises with age, increasing from under two cases per 100 000 population per year in young adults to about 10–20 cases per 100 000 per year over the age of 65 years.

CLINICAL FEATURES

The patient is usually ill, with symptoms present for only a few days or weeks. The most common findings are pallor, fever, various infections and abnormal bleeding. In cases of acute promyelocytic leukaemia (M3), the haemorrhagic manifestations may be particularly severe due to activation of the fibrinolytic and coagulation systems by substances released from cytoplasmic granules. Painful, tender bones are frequently seen in ALL and cause affected children to limp. There may be some enlargement of the liver, spleen and lymph nodes, although these findings are often absent in AML. Particularly in acute myelomonocytic leukaemia (M4) and acute monocytic leukaemia (M5), infiltration of the gums (Fig. 7.1) and skin may be seen. In T-ALL, a mediastinal mass due to thymic enlargement is often found. Symptoms due to meningeal infiltration (headache,

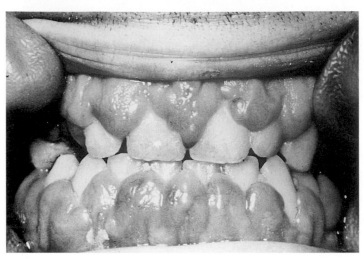

Fig. 7.1 Infiltration of gums by leukaemic cells (monoblasts) in a case of acute monocytic leukaemia.

nausea and vomiting, visual disturbances) are rare at presentation but often develop during the course of acute leukaemia, and particularly of ALL, especially when CNS therapy is not given. Testicular infiltration is also common in treated cases of ALL.

PERIPHERAL BLOOD AND BONE MARROW

A normochromic normocytic anaemia and thrombocytopenia are common. The concentration of white cells in the peripheral blood is usually increased, but this is not an essential feature of leukaemia. About one-third of patients with acute leukaemia have white-cell counts within or even below the normal range ($4-10 \times 10^9/l$) during some stage of the disease, and the remainder have white-cell counts which usually fall in the range $10-50 \times 10^9/l$). The neutrophil count is reduced, often markedly.

In the majority of cases of ALL, a variable proportion of the nucleated cells in the peripheral blood are lymphoblasts. In most patients, the lymphoblasts are small, have little cytoplasm, and are uniform in appearance (FAB category LI; see Table 7.2 and Plate 29), but in others they are larger, with more cytoplasm (L2 and L3; see Table 7.2 and Plate 30). The blood film in AML almost always contains variable numbers of myeloblasts (Fig. 7.2, Plates 31–33). In general, myeloblasts are larger, have more cytoplasm, and are more pleomorphic than lymphoblasts. Furthermore, a proportion of the myeloblasts may contain small numbers of azurophilic cytoplasmic granules, thus indicating their myeloid

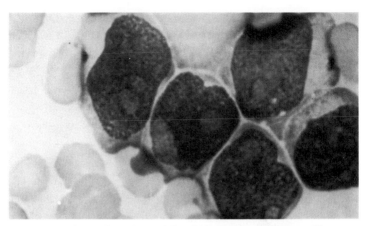

Fig. 7.2 Myeloblasts from the peripheral blood film of a patient with acute myeloid leukaemia. The diameters of these myeloblasts are several times those of adjacent red cells. Their nuclei appear finely stippled and have more than one nucleolus.

lineage (Plate 31). Some of the morphological, cytochemical and immunochemical features that are used to distinguish between leukaemic myeloblasts and lymphoblasts are summarized in Table 7.6. In addition to myeloblasts, other abnormal cells may be found in the blood in AML. These include promyelocytes, myelocytes, agranular neutrophils, neutrophils with the acquired Pelger anomaly (Plate 26), cells of the monocytic series, erythroblasts and megakaryoblasts (see Table 7.1). In occasional patients with acute leukaemia, blast cells may be either absent or difficult to find in the peripheral blood at presentation; such patients are described as having aleukaemic leukaemia.

In both ALL and AML, the bone marrow is usually very hypercellular. In ALL, it is extensively infiltrated with lymphoblasts and lymphocytes. Differences in the morphology of lymphoblasts in the different FAB categories (L1–L3) are given in Table 7.2. In AML, more than 30% of the nucleated marrow cells are leukaemic blasts (usually myeloblasts), or more than 50% are myeloblasts plus promyelocytes. The special cytological features of the bone marrow in different FAB categories of AML (M1–M7) are shown in Table 7.3.

About 25% of adults and 1–4% of children with ALL have the Ph chromosome in their blast cells. Since some patients with chronic granulocytic leukaemia (CGL) may undergo a lymphoblastic transformation and some patients with ALL may develop CGL, it seems that the cell of origin of Ph-positive ALL may be a pluripotent stem cell (i.e. a cell which gives rise both to the lymphoid stem cells and the multipotent

LYMPHOBLASTS AND MYELOBLASTS

	Lymphoblast	Myeloblast
Nucleoli	1–2	2–5
Amount of cytoplasm	Usually scanty	Moderate
Auer rods	Absent	Sometimes present (Plates 34, 35)
Sudan black	Negative	Positive
Peroxidase	Negative	Positive
Periodic-acid-Schiff (PAS)	Positive; large blocks of coarse granules of stained material against a negative background (Plate 36)	Negative or diffuse tinge ± fine granules
Chloroacetate esterase	Negative	Usually positive
Terminal deoxynucleotidyl transferase	Positive	Usually negative
Immunological markers	T-cell lineage markers (e.g. CD2) or B-cell lineage markers (e.g. CD19)	Myeloid lineage markers (e.g. CD13 or CD33)

Table 7.6 Some differences between leukaemic lymphoblasts and myeloblasts.

myeloid stem cells). Ph-negative cases of ALL may have other non-random chromosomal abnormalities. Chromosome abnormalities are also common in the marrow cells of patients with AML and certain abnormalities are uniquely associated with some FAB categories.

TREATMENT

This is based on combinations of cytotoxic drugs and, in some circumstances, allogeneic or autologous bone marrow transplantation. Different cytotoxic regimes are used in ALL and AML. About half of all children with common ALL can be cured with drug schedules including prednisolone and vincristine. By contrast, cytotoxic drugs are much less effective in adults with ALL and in AML. The modes of action of some of the drugs used in the treatment of acute leukaemia are given in Table 7.7. Attempts at killing all leukaemic cells by whole body irradiation

CYTOTOXIC DRUG ACTIONS

Drugs	Mode of action
Prednisolone	Uncertain
Vincristine	Blocks formation of microtubules of the mitotic spindle
Epipodophyllotoxins (etoposide, VP-16)	Interact with topoisomerase II and cause DNA strand breaks
L-Asparaginase	Starves cells of arginine
Methotrexate	Inhibits dihydrofolate reductase and, consequently, thymidylate synthesis
Daunorubicin, hydroxydaunorubicin (Adriamycin)	Intercalate between DNA base pairs and inhibit DNA synthesis
Cytosine arabinoside	Pyrimidine analogue; becomes incorporated into DNA and blocks transcription
Thioguanine, 6-mercaptopurine	Purine analogues; become incorporated into DNA and block transcription

Table 7.7 Modes of action of some cytotoxic drugs used in acute leukaemia.

plus intensive chemotherapy have to be followed by marrow transplantation.

Acute lymphoblastic leukaemia

Therapy with red cell and platelet transfusions and antibiotics may be necessary at presentation. A standard regime for remission induction in children is daunorubicin, L-asparaginase, prednisolone and vincristine. These drugs induce a complete haematological remission in more than 90% of cases overall; the remission rate is nearly 100% in c-ALL but is lower in T-ALL, B-ALL and null-ALL. The same drug regime induces fewer remissions and shorter disease-free survival in adults than in children. The use of different drug combinations in the induction regime improves the remission rate in children with adverse prognostic features and in adults, but may lead to substantial marrow suppression. If severe marrow suppression occurs, intensive support of the type used in AML (see p. 148) will be needed. Patients are also treated with intrathecal methotrexate with or without cranial irradiation to reduce the risk of their developing meningeal leukaemia. In addition, maintenance therapy is carried out for a prolonged period (e.g. 2–3 years) with various cytotoxic drugs in an attempt to kill all residual leukaemic cells. There may also be a place for a short period or periods of intensive chemotherapy with multiple drugs to consolidate the remission. With this type of treatment schedule, about 60% of children with ALL attain long-term disease-free survival and many of these are considered to be cured. With intensive therapy, the proportion of adults attaining long-term disease-free survival is about 35%. A second remission may be induced by chemotherapy in patients who relapse but is short-lived. Those who relapse after a first remission should be considered for transplantation if a second remission can be induced.

Some authorities consider that patients with a white-cell count greater than $50 \times 10^9/l$ or CNS involvement at presentation, those aged less than 2 years or greater than 14 years, and those with B-ALL or certain chromosomal translocations, all of whom have a relatively poor prognosis, should be considered for allogeneic bone marrow transplantation in the first remission. However, it has been argued that even in these patients, comparable leukaemia-free long-term survival could be obtained by transplantation during the second remission (Butturini & Gale 1989).

Acute myeloid leukaemia

A combination of drugs is used to induce remission; drug and dosage schedules are being revised continuously according to empirical observations on their efficacy. An effective combination consists of daunorubicin, cytosine arabinoside and either 6-thioguanine or etoposide. With this type of treatment, prolonged marrow hypoplasia occurs; this is followed by a complete haematological remission in 70–80% of cases under 60 years and 40% of cases over 60 years. The drugs cause severe neutropenia and immunosuppression. Intensive support is required during the phase of marrow hypoplasia, including red cell and platelet transfusions and prophylactic oral antibiotics (to minimize the risk of septicaemia, particularly from the patient's own gut flora). If significant fever develops in a patient with a neutrophil count of less than $0.5 \times 10^9/l$, empiric antibiotic treatment (e.g. with gentamicin and piperacillin intravenously) should be started immediately after taking blood for culture. Successful induction of remission is usually consolidated by a further course or courses of cytotoxic therapy. Maintenance therapy is of doubtful value and is not usually given. The median duration of remission has slowly increased over the years and is now about 2 years, but disease-free long-term survival is seen only in 20–30% of cases under 60 years and 5–15% of cases over 60 years.

In one FAB category of AML known as acute promyelocytic leukaemia (M3) the drug *trans*-retinoic acid induces a remission (p. 141), but the leukaemia relapses rapidly unless consolidation chemotherapy is given.

Allogeneic bone marrow transplantation (p. 158) should be considered in young adults (< 30 years) and children with AML during the first remission. About 40% of patients transplanted in first remission are free of disease at 3 years; since relapse of leukaemia is rare after this time, many of these patients are probably cured. Another effective strategy may be to transplant at first relapse or during a second remission (Butturini & Gale 1989). Autologous marrow transplantation (p. 159) is considered in older patients (who tolerate allogeneic transplantation poorly) and in those without a suitable donor.

Chronic lymphocytic leukaemia (CLL)

This is the commonest form of chronic leukaemia, with an incidence of two to three cases per 100 000 population per year. The male : female ratio is 2 : 1. CLL is rare before the age of 35; over this age, its incidence rises progressively with increasing age. In 98% of cases, the neoplastic clone consists of B-lymphocytes (B-CLL) and in the remainder it consists of T-lymphocytes (T-CLL). Symptoms are not only due to infiltration of the bone marrow and other tissues by the neoplastic cells, but also to a disturbance of both humoral and cellular immunity. There is a reduction in the number of normal B-lymphocytes resulting in a reduced ability to make antibodies. In addition, there is an increase of suppressor T cells and a reduction of helper T cells which probably accounts for the impairment of cell-mediated immunity. Autoimmune phenomena develop in some cases.

CLINICAL FEATURES

Initially CLL is asymptomatic and it is not uncommon for the disease to be discovered accidentally while carrying out a peripheral blood examination for some unrelated reason. Later, the patients are mildly or severely ill and give a history of symptoms that have been present for several months or years. The commonest presenting symptoms are loss of energy, tiredness and shortness of breath. Some patients notice enlargement of superficial lymph nodes. Early in the course of the disease no abnormalities are found on clinical examination. Subsequently, enlargement of the superficial lymph nodes, hepatomegaly and splenomegaly are found. Splenic enlargement is less marked than in chronic myeloid leukaemia, the spleen being rarely enlarged below the level of the umbilicus.

Impairment of humoral immunity and severe neutropenia are present in the later stages of the disease and may cause pneumococcal pneumonia and meningitis and other bacterial infections. The impaired cellular immunity increases susceptibility to infection with *Mycobacterium tuberculosis* and with certain fungi (*Candida*, *Cryptococcus neoformans*) and viruses (herpes zoster, herpes simplex and vaccinia).

Other less common findings include infiltration of the tonsils or skin and Mikulicz's syndrome (enlargement of lachrymal and salivary glands).

PERIPHERAL BLOOD AND BONE MARROW

The essential finding in the peripheral blood is an increase in the lymphocyte count, which may be anywhere between $3.5 \times 10^9/l$ and over $300 \times 10^9/l$; it is usuall greater than $15 \times 10^9/l$. Most of the lymphocytes are mature small lymphocytes (Fig. 7.3, Plate 27). A characteristic feature of the blood film in CLL is the presence of a number of 'smear cells' or 'smudge cells'. These result from an increased mechanical fragility of the neoplastic lymphocytes which are consequently disrupted and squashed

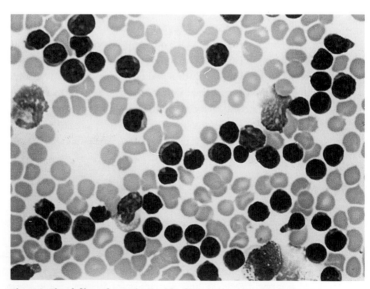

Fig. 7.3 Blood film of a patient with chronic lymphocytic leukaemia (lymphocyte count $300 \times 10^9/l$). There is a marked increase in mature small lymphocytes with scanty cytoplasm and densely-staining nuclei. There are also some smear cells.

during the preparation of blood films. Even when the lymphocytosis is not marked (e.g. below $15 \times 10^9/l$), the diagnosis of CLL can be made by demonstrating that the population of lymphocytes is monoclonal (e.g. by showing that the surface membrane immunoglobulin is of only one light chain type).

Normochromic normocytic anaemia, thrombocytopenia and neutropenia, all due to marrow infiltration, are seen in the later stages of the disease. A positive direct antiglobulin test is found in about 10% of cases and some of these show a mild to severe autoimmune haemolytic anaemia with jaundice, a high reticulocyte count and spherocytosis (p. 67). Some patients may develop autoimmune thrombocytopenic purpura. About 50% of patients with CLL have subnormal IgG, IgA and IgM levels.

Bone marrow aspirates are hypercellular and show varying degrees of infiltration, mainly with mature small lymphocytes but also with larger lymphoid cells. Normal haemopoietic cells may be reduced in number.

PROGRESSION OF CHANGES IN CLL

Dameshek (1967) considered CLL to be a condition in which there was a gradual accumulation of inactive but long-lived lymphocytes. With this concept in mind, Rai et al. (1975) analysed 125 patients and found that four stages in the disease can be characterized, progression from one stage to the next being associated with a shorter life expectation (Table 7.8). Thus, at stage 0 there was only lymphocytosis ($> 15 \times 10^9/l$), and more than 40% of bone marrow cells were lymphocytes; this stage was associated with a median survival of some 10–20 years from the time the stage was diagnosed, the longest lived patient was still alive after 32 years. In stage I, the lymph nodes became palpable and the median survival from

STAGING OF CLL

Stage	Lymphocytosis (blood and marrow)	Enlarged lymph nodes	Enlarged spleen and liver	Anaemia	Thrombo-cytopenia	Median survival (years)
0	*	–	–	–	–	10–20
I	+	*	–	–	–	8
II	+	+/–	*	–	–	6
III	+	+/–	+/–	*	–	1–2
IV	+	+/–	+/–	+/–	*	1–2

Table 7.8 Staging of chronic lymphocytic leukaemia (CLL). The asterisk sign (*) gives the essential feature indicating the stage reached.

then onward was 8 years; stage II was characterized by lymphocytosis with enlargement of the liver or spleen or both, and the median survival was 6 years; stage III was characterized by lymphocytosis and anaemia (Hb concentration < 11 g/dl), and stage IV by lymphocytosis and thrombocytopenia (platelet count < 100 × 10⁹/l); the median survival at stages III and IV was 1–2 years.

Death is often due to causes unrelated to the CLL but may be due to infection complicating neutropenia and immunodeficiency. Rarely, death occurs as a result of malignant transformation. This may be of one of two types:

1 prolymphocytic transformation, in which many of the neoplastic cells in the blood and marrow have the morphology of prolymphocytes rather than small lymphocytes, and

2 lymphomatous transformation (Richter's syndrome), which starts at one site and is manifest by a selective increase in the rate of tumour growth at that site. Eventually, large blast-like cells appear in the circulation and a blood picture resembling that of the leukaemic phase of large cell lymphoma results.

TREATMENT

There is now some evidence that treatment of early disease may *shorten* survival. Consequently, treatment is usually aimed at alleviating symptoms when they develop and at improving bone marrow function when evidence of failure is detected. No treatment is given for stage 0. Stages I and II are only treated if there is bulky lymphadenopathy or if splenomegaly causes discomfort or 'hypersplenism'. The remaining stages are associated with impairment of normal haemopoiesis and must be treated, as must patients with autoimmune haemolytic anaemia or autoimmune thrombocytopenia.

Most patients respond to the alkylating agent chlorambucil either given continuously or in intermittent courses. Cyclophosphamide, another alkylating agent, is also effective. Usually the leukaemia eventually becomes resistant to these drugs. Prednisolone causes a rapid temporary reduction in tumour mass but should not be given for prolonged periods as it increases the chance of infection in an already immunocompromised patient. It is useful in the initial management of autoimmune haemolytic anaemia, autoimmune thrombocytopenia and of marked marrow failure. Recently, the antipurine drug fludarabine has been shown to be very effective against CLL with an overall response rate of 56% in previously treated patients and of 80% in previously untreated patients.

Local radiotherapy is effective in shrinking selected masses of tumour tissue which are causing problems by virtue of their size. It is also of value

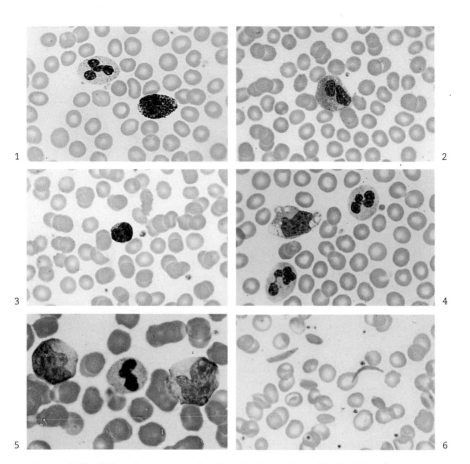

Plates 1–6 Blood films from a normal subject (1–4), a patient with glandular fever (5) and a patient with sickle-cell anaemia (6); May–Grünwald–Giemsa (MGG) stain. (1) Neutrophil granulocyte and basophil granulocyte. (2) Eosinophil granulocyte. (3) Lymphocyte. (4) A monocyte and two neutrophil granulocytes. The monocyte has pale, greyish-blue, vacuolated cytoplasm. (5) Two atypical mononuclear cells and a neutrophil granulocyte from a case of glandular fever. Although the atypical mononuclear cells are similar in size to the monocyte in Plate 4, their cytoplasm is much more basophilic and not vacuolated. (6) Two sickle-shaped and some partially sickled red cells.

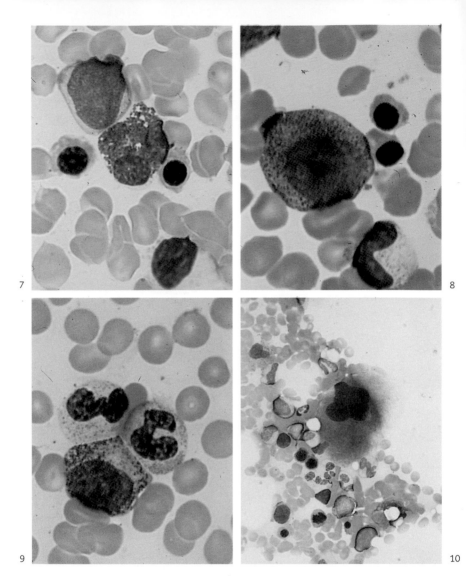

Plates 7–10 Haemopoietic cells from a smear of normal bone marrow (MGG stain). (7) Myeloblast (top left), eosinophil granulocyte (centre) and two late polychromatic normoblasts. (8) Neutrophil promyelocyte, neutrophil metamyelocyte and two late polychromatic normoblasts. (9) Neutrophil myelocyte and two neutrophil band cells. (10) Mature megakaryocyte with granular cytoplasm; this polyploid cell is very large when compared with surrounding diploid bone marrow cells of various types. (Lower magnification than Plates 7–9.)

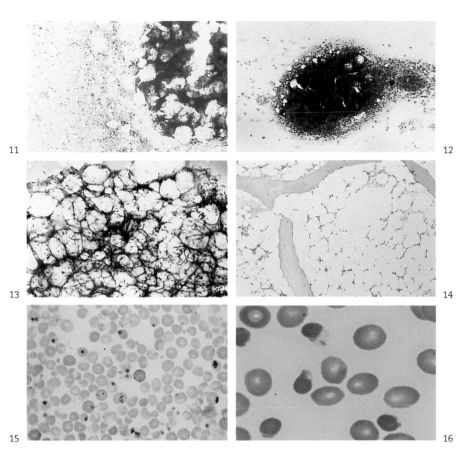

11

12

13

14

15

16

Plates 11–13 Cellularity of marrow fragments in marrow smears from three adult patients (MGG stain). (11) *Normocellular*: about half the volume of the fragment consists of haemopoietic cells (staining blue) and the remainder of unstained rounded, fat cells. (12) *Markedly hypercellular*: virtually all the fat cells are replaced by haemopoietic cells. (13) *Markedly hypocellular*: there are only a few residual haemopoietic cells, most of the fragment consisting of fat cells.

Plate 14 Section of a trephine biopsy of the bone marrow from a patient with aplastic anaemia showing marked hypocellularity (haematoxylin & eosin). Compare with the appearance of the normal trephine biopsy in Fig. 8.5a (p. 170).

Plates 15, 16 (15) Rounded, darkly staining, membrane-bound Heinz bodies consisting of denatured HbH in the red cells of a splenectomized patient with HbH disease (supravital staining with methyl violet). Similar inclusions of denatured HbA may be found in G6PD-deficient patients exposed to oxidant substances. (16) Five 'bite cells' in the blood film of a patient with G6PD deficiency who had received primaquine. These red cells are irregular in shape, abnormally dense and show a poorly staining area just beneath part of the cell membrane (MGG stain).

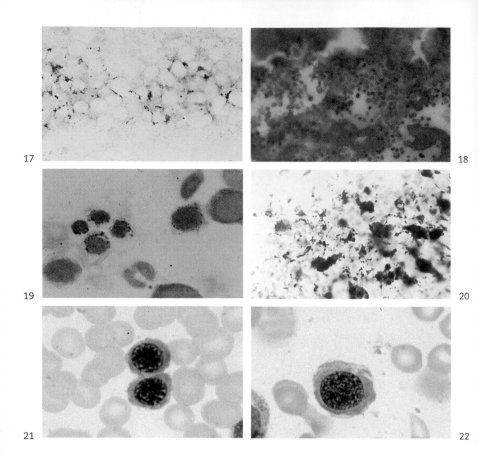

Plates 17–20 Bone marrow smears stained by Perls' acid ferrocyanide method for haemosiderin. (17) Marrow fragment containing normal quantities of storage iron. (18) Marrow fragment from a patient with iron-deficiency anaemia showing an absence of storage iron. (19) Ring sideroblasts from a case of refractory anaemia with ring sideroblasts (primary acquired sideroblastic anaemia). (20) Marrow fragment from a chronically transfused patient with aplastic anaemia, showing a gross excess of storage iron.

Plates 21, 22 (21) Two early polychromatic normoblasts (at centre) from the marrow of a healthy subject. (22) Early polychromatic megaloblast (at centre) from the marrow of an untreated patient with pernicious anaemia. When compared with the early polychromatic normoblasts in Plate 21, the early polychromatic megaloblast is larger and has a more delicate, sieve-like nucleus containing much smaller particles of condensed chromatin. MGG stain.

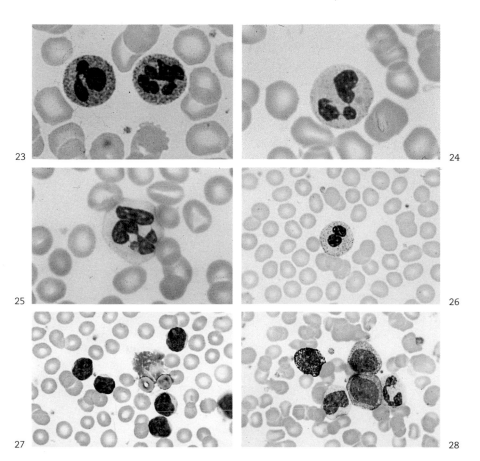

Plates 23–28 Blood films (MGG stain). (23) Toxic granulation in two neutrophil granulocytes from a patient with an infection. (24) Round, pale-blue Döhle body near the nucleus of a neutrophil granulocyte from a patient with extensive burns. Döhle bodies may also be oval or rod-shaped and are more frequently seen at the periphery than at the centre of the cell. (25) Hypogranular neutrophil granulocyte from a patient with a myelodysplastic syndrome. (26) Neutrophil granulocyte from a heterozygote for the inherited Pelger–Huet anomaly. The nucleus is bilobed (spectacle-like) and has markedly condensed chromatin. In heterozygotes for this asymptomatic condition, 50–70% of neutrophil granulocytes show these changes. Similar abnormalities may be found in some neutrophil granulocytes, as an acquired condition, in the myelodysplastic syndromes. (27) Lymphocytes and a smear cell from a case of chronic lymphocytic leukaemia. (28) Two neutrophil myelocytes, a neutrophil metamyelocyte, a neutrophil granulocyte and a basophil from a case of chronic granulocytic leukaemia.

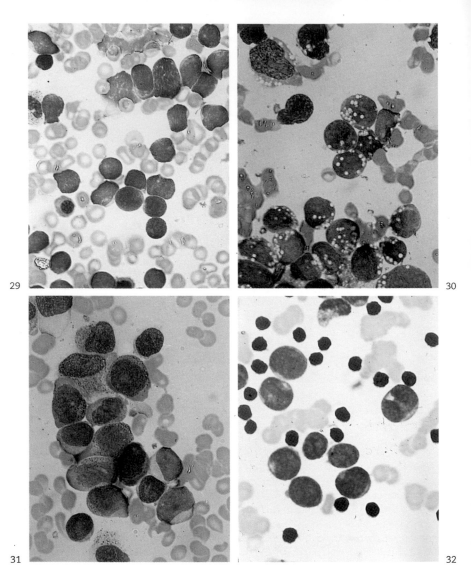

Plates 29–32 Bone marrow smears from patients with acute leukaemia showing infiltration by leukaemic blast cells (MGG stain). (29) Acute lymphoblastic leukaemia, FAB category L1. (30) Acute lymphoblastic leukaemia, FAB category L3; See Table 7.2 on p. 136 for differences from L1 and note prominent cytoplasmic vacuolation. (31) Acute myeloid leukaemia, FAB category M2; note that some of the leukaemic myeloblasts have azurophilic cytoplasmic granules. (32) Combination of acute myeloid leukaemia and chronic lymphocytic leukaemia in the same patient. Note the presence of two populations of leukaemic cells, the myeloblasts of acute myeloid leukaemia and the much smaller lymphocytes of chronic lymphocytic leukaemia.

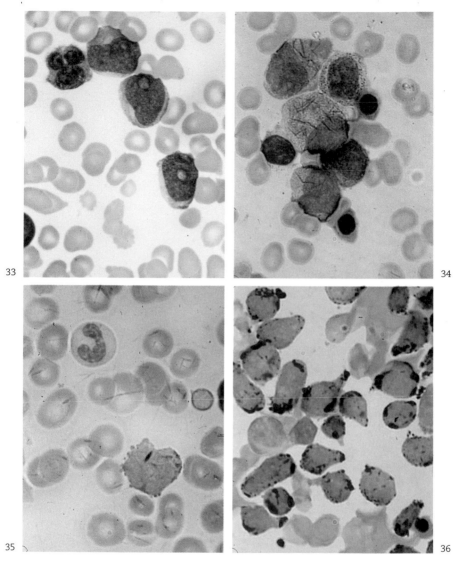

Plates 33–36 Bone marrow smears from patients with acute leukaemia. (33) Acute myeloid leukaemia (FAB category M1); the three leukaemic myeloblasts show prominent nucleoli. MGG stain. (34) Myeloblasts of acute myeloid leukaemia showing several Auer rods (MGG stain). These are azurophilic needle-shaped or rod-shaped intracytoplasmic inclusions which are exclusively found in some of the leukaemic myeloblasts of a small proportion of patients with acute myeloid leukaemia or chronic myeloid leukaemia in blast cell transformation. (35) Leukaemic myeloblasts reacted with Sudan black (which stains azurophilic granules), showing positive staining of Auer rods. (36) Acute lymphoblastic leukaemia; the smear has been stained by the Periodic acid-Schiff reaction for glycogen and shows large positively stained blocks in the cytoplasm of the leukaemic lymphoblasts.

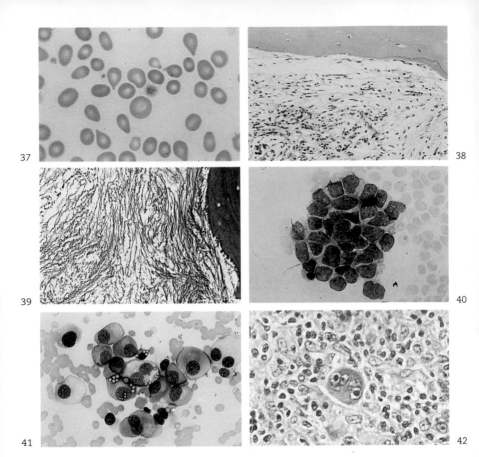

Plates 37–42 (37) Blood film of a patient with idiopathic myelofibrosis showing several tear-drop-shaped poikilocytes and an abnormally large platelet. MGG stain. (38) Trephine biopsy of the bone marrow of a patient with idiopathic myelofibrosis showing fibroblasts and collagen fibrosis (haematoxylin & eosin). (39) Section of the same trephine biopsy showing increased reticulin fibres (silver impregnation of reticulin). (40) Clump of metastatic tumour cells in a marrow smear (MGG stain). (41) Marrow smear from a patient with multiple myeloma (MGG stain). (42) Lymph node of a patient with Hodgkin's disease showing a large multinucleate Reed–Sternberg cell at the centre (haematoxylin & eosin).

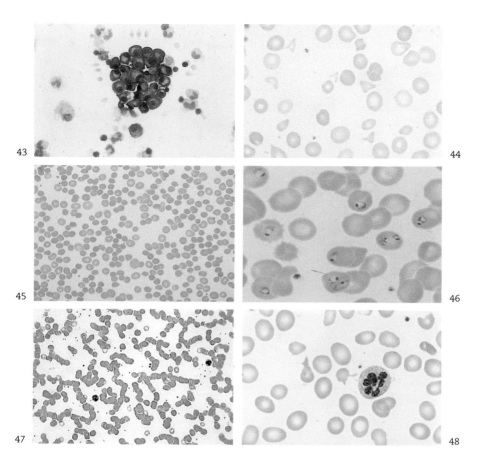

Plates 43–48 (43) Marrow smear showing myeloma cells reacting with antibody against λ-chains; the reaction was demonstrated using an immunoalkaline phosphatase method. The cells did not react with antibody against κ-chains and were, therefore, monoclonal in origin. The serum contained an IgD λ paraprotein. (44) Fragmented red cells (schistocytes) in the blood film of a patient with a malfunctioning aortic valve prosthesis. MGG stain. (45) Blood film from a patient with hereditary spherocytosis showing spherocytes (MGG stain). (46) Blood smear from a patient with *Plasmodium falciparum* malaria showing several parasitized red cells (MGG stain). The parasites appear as small rings with one or two chromatin dots. (47) Blood film from a patient with multiple myeloma showing marked red-cell rouleaux formation (MGG stain). (48) Blood smear from a patient with severe pernicious anaemia showing a hypersegmented neutrophil granulocyte, oval macrocytes and other poikilocytes (MGG stain).

in the management of hypersplenism when the splenomegaly does not respond to chemotherapy. Infections should be treated vigorously when they occur. Patients with recurrent infections are helped by regular intravenous gamma-globulin therapy.

Prolymphocytic leukaemia (PLL)

This is a disease, mainly affecting the elderly, caused by a monoclonal proliferation of prolymphocytes. These cells are more mature than the lymphoblasts of ALL but less mature than the lymphocytes of CLL. Typically the prolymphocytes are larger than lymphocytes, with more abundant cytoplasm, a less condensed chromatin pattern and prominent nucleoli. In about 80% of cases, the malignant cells belong to the B-cell lineage and in the remainder to the T-cell lineage. PLL is commonest in the elderly and is characterized by:

1 considerable splenomegaly;
2 very high white blood cell count (WBC), usually $>100 \times 10^9/l$, the majority of which are prolymphocytes;
3 little lymph node enlargement (except in T-PLL);
4 skin infiltration (only in T-PLL), and
5 poorer response to chemotherapy than CLL.

Hairy cell leukaemia

This is an uncommon disease with a peak incidence in the sixth decade and a strong male preponderance. It is caused by a monoclonal proliferation of cells with thread-like cytoplasmic processes at their surface (hairy cells). These cells may be infrequent in the blood but are usually readily found in the bone marrow and spleen. In most cases, the hairy cells belong to the B-cell lineage. The main features of the disease are:

1 moderate splenomegaly;
2 pancytopenia due to
   (a) infiltration of the marrow by hairy cells and
   (b) hypersplenism;
3 hairy cells in the blood and marrow;
4 variable clinical course often with survival for many years without specific therapy, and
5 striking response to prolonged treatment with α-interferon, the adenosine deaminase inhibitor deoxycoformycin or the antipurine chlordeoxyadenosine.

Chronic granulocytic leukaemia (CGL) (chronic myeloid leukaemia)

The incidence of this form of chronic leukaemia is about 1 per 100 000 population per year. The disease is rare in children; its incidence in adults rises steadily with increasing age. The Ph chromosome (p. 140) is present in over 95% of the cases, not only in neutrophil precursors but also in erythroblasts, megakaryocytes and some B-lymphocytes. The malignant clone appears to arise from a pluripotent haemopoietic stem cell.

CLINICAL FEATURES

Most patients are symptomatic at the time of diagnosis. Common symptoms are low-grade fever, anorexia, weight loss and night sweats (due to a raised metabolic rate), lassitude, dyspnoea and palpitations (due to anaemia), discomfort over the left side of the abdomen (due to massive splenomegaly) and bruising and other haemorrhagic manifestations (due to abnormalities in the number and function of platelets). Rarer symptoms seen in patients with WBC $> 500 \times 10^9/l$ are headaches, dizziness, tinnitus, deafness, ataxia and even coma; these result from impairment of cerebral blood flow due to increased blood viscosity as well as from vascular obstruction by leucocytes. Priapism is also seen occasionally and may have the same basis. Gout and uric acid stones may result from hyperuricaemia due to increased nucleic acid turnover.

PERIPHERAL BLOOD AND BONE MARROW

The blood count often shows a normochromic normocytic anaemia. The white cell count is elevated, usually to between $50 \times 10^9/l$ and $400 \times 10^9/l$. The platelet count is often high, but may be normal or low. Most of the white cells consist of *neutrophil granulocytes*, band cells, metamyelocytes and *myelocytes* (see Figs 7.4 and 7.5, Plate 28). Blast cells account for a relatively small proportion of the leucocytes. There is virtually always an increase in the absolute basophil count and, commonly, an increase in the absolute eosinophil and monocyte counts. Megakaryocytes may be seen in the blood film. The neutrophil alkaline phosphatase score is reduced in about 90% of patients. There is an increase in the serum vitamin B_{12} concentration and the serum vitamin B_{12} binding capacity, due to increased production of transcobalamin I, a B_{12}-carrying protein released by granulocytes and their precursors.

The bone marrow is extremely hypercellular. There is hyperplasia of the neutrophil, eosinophil and basophil granulocyte series and an increase in megakaryocytes. In the chronic phase of the disease, less than 15% of

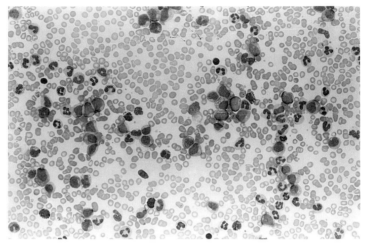

Fig. 7.4 Blood film of a patient with chronic granulocytic leukaemia. The total white-cell count is markedly increased (200 × 10⁹/l) and the majority of the white cells consists of neutrophil granulocytes, band cells, metamyelocytes and myelocytes.

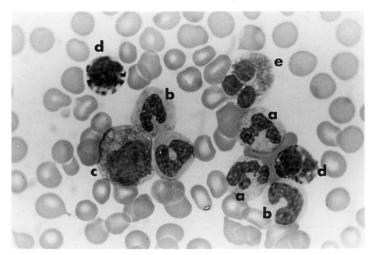

Fig. 7.5 Higher power view of some of the white cells from the blood film shown in Fig. 7.4. (a) Neutrophil granulocytes; (b) neutrophil metamyelocytes; (c) neutrophil myelocyte; (d) basophil granulocytes; and (e) eosinophil granulocyte.

nucleated marrow cells are blast cells. Trephine biopsies may show some increase in reticulin.

PROGRESSION OF CHANGES IN CGL

Detailed follow-up studies of the survivors of the atomic bomb explosions in Japan in 1945 have elucidated the pattern of progression of changes in CGL (Kamada & Uchino 1978). The appearance of the Ph chromosome is probably the first manifestation of the disease. The earliest change in the peripheral blood is an increase of the leucocyte count above the upper limit of normal (11 $\times$ 10^9/l). At the same time, basophilia, thrombocytosis and the low neutrophil alkaline phosphatase make their appearance. As the count rises to 20 $\times$ 10^9/l, the percentage of neutrophil precursors in the peripheral blood rises above 5% of the total white-cell count and the increase in serum vitamin B$_{12}$ becomes apparent. Splenomegaly is found when the count is in the region of 50 $\times$ 10^9/l and shortly after that, symptoms arise. It has been calculated that if all the leukaemic cells were derived from a single cell with a Ph chromosome, then it would take about 6 years for the leucocyte count to reach about 100 $\times$ 10^9/l. The leucocyte count in CGL increases with time and the rate of increase is exponential; that is, the number doubles at regular intervals. The actual interval in which doubling takes place varies between patients, and is often over 70 days. The increase in total leucocyte count is accompanied by an increase in the size of the spleen and by a fall in Hb concentration.

Metamorphosis of CGL (acute-phase transformation)

All patients with chronic granulocytic leukaemia develop a more rapidly progressive terminal phase, although the exact form that this takes shows considerable variation between patients. The metamorphosis is the consequence of the evolution from the original Ph-positive clone of a new clone of leukaemic cells which is more malignant than the parent clone. The new clone, which may have additional chromosome abnormalities, either originates in an extramedullary site and subsequently spreads to the blood and marrow, or originates in the bone marrow and spreads rapidly into the blood and other tissues. The cells which accumulate in acute-phase transformation are usually myeloblasts, but in a third of patients they are lymphoblasts (blast-cell transformation or blast crisis). Occasionally, they may be neutrophil promyelocytes, monoblasts, basophil or mast-cell precursors, megakaryocytes or erythroblasts. The clinical features of transformation include fever, malaise, loss of weight, night sweats, bone pain, a rapidly enlarging spleen or extramedullary tumour mass, and resistance to standard therapy.

TREATMENT

Treatment (Kantarjian et al. 1993) is aimed at: (a) reducing the leucocyte count to normal limits, as this is followed by a marked alleviation of symptoms and a rise in Hb concentration; and (b) the more difficult task of eliminating the neoplastic clone.

The current drugs of choice are α-interferon (up to 3×10^6 units s.c. daily) or hydroxyurea (0.5–3.0 g daily by mouth); interferons are naturally occurring biological response modifiers and hydroxyurea acts by inhibiting ribonucleotide reductase and, consequently, impairing DNA synthesis. The alkylating agent busulphan is as effective as hydroxyurea but is more toxic. With α-interferon, a complete haematological response is seen in 70–80% of cases, and a major cytogenetic response (i.e. proportion of Ph-positive metaphases reduced to <35%) in 30–40%. Side-effects of fever, chills, post-nasal drip and anorexia are seen in most patients but can be managed with paracetamol. More serious side-effects include depression, fatigue and insomnia (which respond to antidepressants), and immune-mediated tissue damage. Hydroxyurea or busulphan, when used on their own, also cause a complete haematological remission in 70–80% of cases but greater than 90% of metaphases remain Ph-positive in virtually all cases (i.e. the haematological response is a pseudo-remission not a true remission). Busulphan may be administered continuously until the leucocyte count falls to about $20 \times 10^9/l$. If the busulphan is then stopped, the leucocyte count will continue to fall for a few weeks and then start to rise. When the increase in cell count is relatively slow, busulphan can be given intermittently, recommencing therapy when the white-cell count rises to around $50 \times 10^9/l$. However, if the white-cell count increases rapidly, a small maintenance dose may be given continuously. Busulphan may cause side-effects such as pulmonary fibrosis, skin pigmentation and aplasia of the marrow.

Irrespective of which drug is used, it is customary also to administer 300 mg allopurinol daily during the early phases of treatment, to prevent marked increases in the uric acid level as a consequence of the destruction of tumour cells.

If symptoms related to hyperviscosity of the blood and leucocyte-related vasular obstruction are present in patients with very high white-cell counts, the counts should be rapidly reduced by repeated leucapheresis and high doses of hydroxyurea.

The median survival of patients treated with α-interferon is 6 years and of patients treated with hydroxyurea or busulphan is 4 years. Some patients survive for as long as 10–15 years. When the treatment includes α-interferon, 50–60% are alive at 5 years. Once metamorphosis occurs, the outlook is bad; the majority of patients die within 1–2 months.

One form of treatment for patients under the age of 50 who have an HLA-compatible sibling is allogeneic bone marrow transplantation in the chronic phase, within 1 year of diagnosis. This procedure provides a 40–60% chance of cure, but carries a substantial morbidity and mortality; the main causes of death are graft-versus-host disease, interstitial pneumonitis or both. The value of high-dose chemotherapy or radiation therapy in the chronic phase, followed by autologous bone marrow or peripheral-blood-derived stem-cell transplantation (p. 14) is currently being investigated.

Bone marrow transplantation

The possiblility of bone marrow transplantation (BMT) allows the dose of chemotherapy or radiotherapy or both to be escalated to such an extent that there is a substantial chance of completely eliminating the leukaemic cells (i.e. of curing the patient). The BMT rescues the patient from the marrow failure that inevitably follows such intensive therapy; without BMT such therapy would be uniformly fatal. The intensive chemotherapy plus or minus total body irradiation ensures that autologous bone marrow reconstitution is unlikely and also causes immunosuppression, thus permitting successful engraftment. Donor marrow is obtained from an HLA-matched and mixed-lymphocyte-culture-compatible sibling or, when this is not possible, from an HLA-matched unrelated individual (allogeneic BMT). The donor marrow is harvested under general or spinal anaesthesia by multiple aspirations from the iliac crests and infused intravenously into the recipient. The injected pluripotent haemopoietic stem cells circulate and seed the recipient's bone marrow stroma. Monocytes and neutrophils appear in the blood after 2–3 weeks followed by platelets and red cells.

The problems associated with allogeneic transplantation are: failure to engraft or, rarely, rejection following engraftment; acute and chronic graft-versus-host disease and recurrence of leukaemia. There is an early transplant-related mortality (up to 10–15%) which is largely due to infection (including cytomegalovirus interstitial pneumonitis).

Allogeneic transplantation has a place in the management not only of acute myeloid, acute lymphoblastic and chronic myeloid leukaemia, but also in severe aplastic anaemia and some inherited disorders such as severe combined immunodeficiency disease, chronic granulomatous disease of childhood, Chediak–Higashi syndrome, Fanconi's anaemia, Hurler's disease and Gaucher's disease. Cures have also been reported in children with sickle-cell anaemia and homozygous β-thalassaemia.

Allogeneic transplants have been performed in leukaemia mostly in patients under 50 years. Some leukaemia centres perform autologous BMT in older patients or when a compatible sibling donor is not available. In this procedure, the patient's own marrow is aspirated and cryopreserved during the first remission. When the patient relapses, chemoradiotherapy is given and the stored marrow is used to reconstitute haemopoiesis, sometimes after purging residual leukaemic cells *in vitro* using antibodies or drugs. Autologous transplantation has also been used after escalated doses of chemotherapy, to repopulate the marrow in patients with lymphoma (usually after the first relapse), myeloma and tumours of non-haemopoietic tissue (e.g. carcinoma of the breast).

It has now been established that following ablation, the marrow can be repopulated not only with intravenous infusions of bone marrow cells but also of peripheral blood-derived stem cells.

References

Bennett J.M., Catovsky D., Daniel M.T., Flandrin G., Galton D.A.G., Gralnick H.R., Sultan C. (1976) Proposals for the classification of the acute leukaemias. *Br. J. Haematol.* **33**, 451–458.

Bennett J.M., Catovsky D., Daniel M.T., Flandrin G., Galton D.A.G., Gralnick H.R., Sultan C. (1980) A variant form of hypergranular promyelocytic leukaemia (M3). *Br J. Haematol.* **44**, 169–170.

Butturini A., Gale R.P. (1989) Annotation: chemotherapy versus transplantation in acute leukaemia. *Br. J. Haematol.* **72**, 1–8.

Cartwright R.A., Staines A. (1992) Acute leukaemias. *Clin. Haematol.* **5**, 1–26.

Cline M.J. (1994) The molecular basis of leukemia. *New Engl. J. Med.* **330**, 328–336.

Dameshek W. (1967) Chronic lymphocytic leukemia–an accumulative disease of immunologically incompetent lymphocytes. *Blood* **29**, 566–584.

Kamada N., Uchino H. (1978) Chronological sequence of appearance of clinical and laboratory findings characteristic of chronic myelocytic leukemia. *Blood* **51**, 843–850.

Kantarjian H.M., Deisseroth A., Kurzrock R., Estrov Z., Talpaz M. (1993) Chronic myelogenous leukemia: a concise update. *Blood* **82**, 691–703.

Rai K.R., Sawitsky A., Cronkite E.P., Chanana A.D., Levy R.N., Pasternak B.S. (1975) Clinical staging of chronic lymphocytic leukemia. *Blood* **46**, 219–234.

Reviews

Canellos G.P. (ed.) (1990) Chronic leukemias. *Hematol./Oncol. Clin. N. Am.* **4**, 319–502.

Catovsky D., Foa R. (1990) *The Lymphoid Leukaemias.* Butterworth, London.

Finch S.C., Linet M.S. (1992) Chronic leukaemias. *Clin. Haematol.* **5**, 27–56.

Hughes T.P., Goldman J.M. (1991) Chronic myeloid leukaemia. In: Hoffman R., Benz E.J., Shattil S.J., Furie B., Cohen H.J. (eds.) *Hematology: Basic Principles and Practice*, pp 854–869. Churchill Livingstone, New York.

Hoelzer D. (ed.) (1994) *Acute Lymphoblastic Leukaemia.* Baillière's Clinical Haematology.

International Practice and Research, Vol 7/No 2. Baillière Tindall, London.

Rozman C. (ed.) (1993) *Chronic Lymphocytic Leukaemia and Related Disorders.* Baillière's Clinical Haematology. International Practice and Research, Vol 6/No 4. Baillière Tindall, London.

Whittaker J.A. (ed.) (1992) *Leukaemia,* 2nd edn. Blackwell Scientific Publications, Oxford.

Young B.D. (ed.) (1992) *The Molecular Genetics of Haematological Malignancy.* Baillière's Clinical Haematology. International Practice and Research, Vol 5/No 4. Baillière Tindall, London.

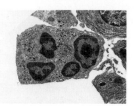

Chronic Myeloproliferative Disorders

Objectives in learning

1   To know the features common to this group of disorders.
2   To know the pathogenesis, clinical and laboratory manifestations and the natural history of the four main chronic myeloproliferative disorders and current approaches to therapy.
3   To understand the differential diagnosis of polycythaemia, a high platelet count and myelofibrosis.

The chronic myeloproliferative disorders are a group of related conditions characterized by the proliferation of a neoplastic clone of low malignancy derived from a pluripotent or multipotent haemopoietic stem cell. The four conditions which are included under this heading are polycythaemia rubra vera; essential thrombocythaemia; idiopathic myelofibrosis; and chronic granulocytic leukaemia (Rosenthal 1992). Some authors exclude chronic granulocytic leukaemia from this group but there is no valid reason for doing so, there being no fundamental difference between the chronic phase of chronic granulocytic leukaemia and the three other conditions. Although many patients with a chronic myeloproliferative disorder can be classified into the four conditions at diagnosis, there are a number of unclassifiable patients with intermediate characteristics who clearly belong in this group. Except in idiopathic myelofibrosis, the abnormal clone generates increased concentrations of one or more of the following cell types in the peripheral blood: erythrocytes, platelets, granulocytes and monocytes. Some patients with polycythaemia rubra vera and essential thrombocythaemia, and occasional patients with chronic granulocytic leukaemia, develop extensive myelofibrosis during the course of their illness. The fibroblasts responsible for the myelofibrosis in these conditions as well as in idiopathic myelofibrosis do not belong to the neoplastic clone; the fibrosis seems to result from the release of fibroblast-stimulating factors by abnormal megakaryocytes (i.e. the fibrosis is reactive). Another common feature of the chronic myeloproliferative disorders is that they may all terminate in acute leukaemia. Treatment of these disorders is usually aimed not at cure but at alleviating symptoms and reducing the risk of serious complications; however, some patients with chronic granulocytic leukaemia may be cured by marrow transplantation (p. 158).

The myelodysplastic syndromes resemble the chronic myeloproliferative disorders in resulting from the proliferation of an abnormal clone of low malignancy derived from a haemopoietic stem cell. The distinction between the two types of disease is based on the finding of disordered maturation of blood cells (dysplasia) at presentation in the former but not the latter.

Since a progressive and marked increase in the leucocyte count is the most striking haematological feature of chronic granulocytic leukaemia, this disorder is discussed in the section on leukaemia on p. 154 rather than in this chapter.

Polycythaemia rubra vera (Primary proliferative polycythaemia)

Polycythaemia rubra vera (Landaw 1990) is a chronic disease in which there is a slowly expanding mutant cell clone derived from a multipotent haemopoietic stem cell. The mutant clone gives rise to increased numbers of red cells and, often, of neutrophils and platelets. The erythroid progenitor cells (p. 14) derived from the clone are abnormal in that they form colonies *in vitro* in the presence of only trace quantities of erythropoietin (i.e. they are abnormally sensitive to erythropoietin). The clonal nature of the abnormal cell population has been shown by the demonstration that in women with polycythaemia rubra vera who are heterozygous at the X-chromosome-linked locus for glucose-6-phosphate dehydrogenase (G6PD), the red cells, granulocytes and platelets contain only one of the two isoenzyme types, whereas cells unaffected by the disease (e.g. skin fibroblasts) contain both. Most of the symptoms and complications of the disease can be attributed to the high red-cell count and packed cell volume (PCV) which causes an increase in blood volume and viscosity. The latter leads to decreased blood flow through the tissues.

CLINICAL FEATURES

Patients are usually aged between 40 and 70 years. In the early stages of the disease there may be no symptoms and a raised haemoglobin (Hb) concentration may be an incidental finding. Symptoms are often insidious in onset and numerous. They include headache, weakness, generalized pruritus, dizziness, sweating, visual disturbances, weight loss and dyspnoea on exertion. Some patients present acutely with a thrombotic or haemorrhagic episode.

Venous thromboses and superficial thrombophlebitis are more common than arterial thromboses. There may be thrombosis of deep veins (sometimes with embolism), or of mesenteric, splenic, portal or hepatic veins. Arterial thromboses may cause cerebral or cardiac infarcts or peripheral gangrene (Fig. 8.1). In Videbaek's series from Copenhagen (Videbaek 1950), nearly one-third of the patients had thrombotic episodes and these accounted for 20% of the deaths. The incidence of vascular occlusion has been found to be correlated directly with the PCV (Pearson & Wetherley-Mein 1978). Patients with a PCV greater than 0.6 have occlusive episodes at a rate of almost one each year (Fig. 8.2). The risk of vascular occlusion may be greater in patients with high platelet counts than in those with normal counts.

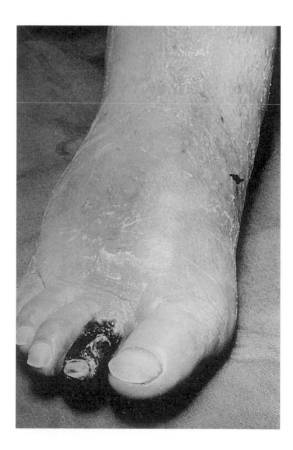

Fig. 8.1 Gangrene of a toe in a patient with polycythaemia rubra vera.

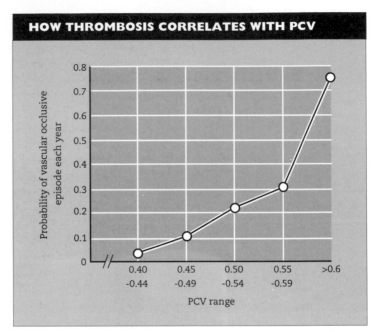

Fig. 8.2 The probability of the occurrence of a vascular occlusive episode related to the PCV. A probability of 0.1 indicates a 1 in 10 chance of the occurrence (after Pearson & Wetherley-Mein 1978).

Some patients have peptic ulcers and may bleed from them, but there is uncertainty as to whether the incidence of peptic ulceration is greater than in the normal population. About 10% of cases suffer from gout secondary to increased haemopoietic activity leading to an increase in nucleic acid turnover and uric acid production.

Haemorrhagic manifestations may also occur and include ecchymoses, epistaxis and life-threatening intra- and post-operative bleeding. The cause of the bleeding is not well understood. It may be related to the presence of abnormally large platelets with various biochemical and functional defects (e.g. abnormal membrane glycoprotein patterns, lipoxygenase deficiency, acquired storaged pool disease and altered response to aggregating agents such as ADP, see pp. 206, 214).

On examination, there may be a florid dusky-red colour of the face, lips, hands and feet, congestion of the conjunctival vessels and marked distension of retinal veins. Splenomegaly, usually of moderate degree, is seen in about 70% of patients at presentation. The liver is enlarged in half the cases.

LABORATORY FINDINGS

The Hb concentration, red-cell count and PCV are high; Hb values of 18–24 g/dl are common and the PCV is usually well over 0.47 in females and 0.52 in males. The total red-cell volume (measured using ^{51}Cr-labelled red cells) is increased, indicating the presence of true polycythaemia. The total plasma volume (measured using ^{125}I-labelled albumin) is usually decreased or normal and the total blood volume is increased. The red cells are usually normochromic and normocytic. However, they may be hypochromic and microcytic due to absolute or relative iron deficiency. A true iron deficiency may result from recurrent spontaneous gastrointestinal haemorrhage and repeated venesection. A relative iron deficiency arises from the inability of a normal store of body iron to meet the needs of a markedly expanded red-cell renewal system. Other haematological features are:

1 neutrophil leucocytosis (usually up to 30 × 10^9/l) in 75% of cases, often with some metamyelocytes and myelocytes on the blood film;

2 raised or normal neutrophil leucocyte alkaline phosphatase score;

3 increased absolute basophil count in some cases;

4 raised platelet count (up to 1000 × 10^9/l or higher) in two-thirds of the cases;

5 elevated serum vitamin B$_{12}$ level due to an increase in transcobalamin I;

6 increased whole blood viscosity;

7 decreased plasma and urinary erythropoietin levels;

8 hyperuricaemia in 70% of patients, and

9 various cytogenetic abnormalities in the bone marrow cells of about 30% of newly-diagnosed patients, including extra chromosomes 8 and 9 and structural abnormalities of chromosome 20.

In most cases, marrow smears and trephine biopsies show an increase in cellularity, with a corresponding reduction in fat cells. The increased cellularity is caused by hyperplasia, particularly of the erythropoietic cells but also of the granulocytopoietic cells and megakaryocytes.

DIFFERENTIAL DIAGNOSIS

Other causes of true polycythaemia (i.e. causes of secondary polycythaemia, see p. 33) must be excluded by appropriate investigations (e.g. sonography to exclude renal lesions). A definite diagnosis of polycythaemia rubra vera may be made when an increase in red-cell mass is associated with normal arterial O$_2$ saturation and either splenomegaly or at least two of the following: neutrophil leucocytosis; thrombocytosis; high neutrophil alkaline phosphatase score; and elevated serum vitamin B$_{12}$ level. When the increased red-cell mass is not associated with these diagnostic features (and secondary polycythaemia has been excluded), the condition is best described as idiopathic erythrocytosis. On prolonged follow-up, some patients with idiopathic erythrocytosis eventually develop the full-blown picture of polycythaemia rubra vera, but others do not.

TREATMENT AND PROGNOSIS

The aim of treatment is to maintain the PCV below 0.50, and preferably below 0.45, thus preventing dangerous thrombotic episodes (see Fig. 8.2). Venesection relieves symptoms rapidly and is the treatment of choice in the first instance. If long-term control of the PCV requires frequent venesections (e.g. more than once every 2 months) or if there is a substantial thrombocytosis (venesection may actually increase the thrombocytosis), myelosuppressive treatment with hydroxyurea (Löfzenberg & Wahlin 1988), busulphan or irradiation of the bone marrow using an intravenous injection of radioactive phosphorus (^{32}P) (which is incorporated into bone) should be instituted; hydroxyurea is the drug of choice in patients under 60 years of age since it appears to be non-leukaemogenic. A single injection of ^{32}P often controls both the high PCV and high platelet count for more than a year. Further injections may be given when necessary (Fig. 8.3).

The median survival from diagnosis is 18 months in untreated patients and 10–16 years in patients adequately treated with venesection alone, venesection plus either hydroxyurea or an alkylating agent, or venesection plus ^{32}P. The main causes of death in treated patients are thrombosis and acute leukaemia; thrombotic deaths are more common in patients treated with venesection only than in other patients. The incidence of terminal acute leukaemia is higher in patients treated with ^{32}P (about 10%) and alkylating agents than in those treated with venesection alone (2–4%) or hydroxyurea. The clinicopathological picture of idiopathic myelofibrosis develops in 10–25% of cases. There is now some evidence that the development of myelofibrosis is delayed by 4 or 5 years if myelosuppressive therapy is used, presumably because this causes a reduction in the number of abnormal megakaryocytes in the marrow (p. 161).

Essential thrombocythaemia

This chronic myeloproliferative disorder (Tobelem 1989; Tefferi & Hoagland 1994) is usually seen in middle-aged or elderly individuals and is closely related to polycythaemia rubra vera. It is characterized by:

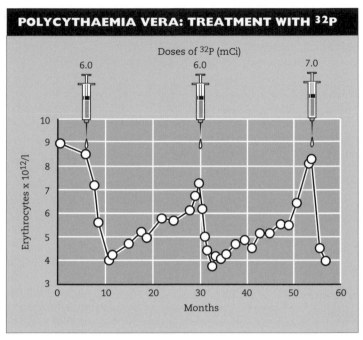

Fig. 8.3 The effect of giving three doses of ^{32}P on the erythrocyte count of a patient with polycythaemia vera (after Szur et al. 1959).

1   recurrent bleeding due to abnormal platelet function (e.g. gastro-intestinal haemorrhage, haematuria and bruising);
2   episodes of both arterial and venous thrombosis;
3   a platelet count persistently greater than $600 \times 10^9/l$ (usually in the range $1000-4000 \times 10^9/l$);
4   some abnormally large platelets with bizarre shapes, and
5   a hypercellular bone marrow with a marked increase in the number of megakaryocytes and abnormally large megakaryocytes.
G6PD isoenzyme studies have shown that the platelets are derived from a single mutant cell clone. There is often a moderate neutrophil leucocytosis and a basophilia. The Hb concentration is either normal or slightly increased. Iron-deficiency anaemia due to chronic gastrointestinal blood loss may develop, and the serum uric acid level may be raised. Thrombotic episodes are seen more frequently in older patients and are presumably caused by a combination of the very high platelet count and degenerative vascular disease. The spleen is enlarged early in the disease

CAUSES OF THROMBOCYTOSIS

Reactive
Haemorrhage, haemolysis, trauma, surgery, post-partum, recovery from
  thrombocytopenia
Acute and chronic infections
Chronic inflammatory disease (e.g. ulcerative colitis, rheumatoid
  arthritis)
Malignant disease (e.g. carcinoma, Hodgkin's disease)
Splenectomy and splenic atrophy
Iron-deficiency anaemia

Chronic myeloproliferative disorders
Essential thrombocythaemia, polycythaemia rubra vera, chronic
  granulocytic leukaemia, idiopathic myelofibrosis

Table 8.1

but eventually undergoes atrophy from repeated infarction. The disease
runs a chronic course and evolves into either myelofibrosis in about 10%
of cases or acute leukaemia in about 5%.

The differential diagnosis includes other chronic myeloproliferative
disorders and a reactive thrombocytosis (Table 8.1).

There is no clear evidence yet that asymptomatic patients with
thrombocytosis benefit from lowering the platelet count although there
is an expectation that this should be so. In patients with a history of
haemorrhage or thrombosis, hydroxyurea (by mouth) (Löfzenberg &
Wahlin 1988) or α-interferon (by s.c. injection) (Talpaz et al. 1989) is
used. Some clinicians use the same treatment in young, asymptomatic
patients with a platelet count more than $1000 \times 10^9/l$, or in elderly
asymptomatic patients. The aim of therapy is to reduce the platelet
count to below $500 \times 10^9/l$ and so prevent thrombotic and
haemorrhagic complications. Low-dose busulphan or ^{32}P are also effective but are now less commonly used than previously because of
the long-term risk of leukaemogenesis. Some physicians use low-dose
aspirin, in the hope of reducing the risk of thrombosis in asymptomatic
young patients (e.g. <50 years) with platelets counts less than $1000 \times
10^9/l$. Symptoms such as intermittent digital ischaemia and transient
cerebral ischaemic attacks may respond to inhibitors of platelet aggregation such as aspirin and dipyridamole; however, since platelet function
is abnormal in this condition, these drugs could increase the risk of
haemorrhage.

Idiopathic myelofibrosis (myelosclerosis, agnogenic myeloid metaplasia)

Studies using G6PD isoenzyme markers and cytogenetic markers have confirmed the presence in idiopathic myelofibrosis of a neoplastic clone derived from a multipotent haemopoietic stem cell. The fibroblasts found in the bone marrow are not part of the abnormal clone. It is thought that the neoplastic clone generates abnormal megakaryocytes which cause the fibrosis by releasing platelet-derived growth factor which stimulates fibroblast proliferation and platelet factor 4 which inhibits collagenase.

Idiopathic myelofibrosis (Weinstein 1991; Hasselbach 1993) is a chronic disorder usually found between the ages of 40 and 70 years. Its main features are:

1 moderate to gross splenomegaly (Fig. 8.4), sometimes causing abdominal discomfort;

2 constitutional symptoms such as anorexia, weight loss, fever and night sweats (usually in the later stages of the disease);

3 a leucoerythroblastic anaemia (p. 131);

4 the presence of many tear-drop-shaped poikilocytes in the blood film (Plate 37);

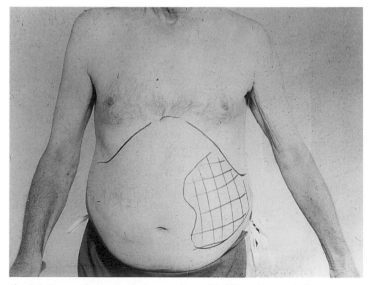

Fig. 8.4 Gross splenomegaly in a patient with idiopathic myelofibrosis.

5   progressive fibrosis of the marrow and, in some cases, a thickening of the bone trabeculae (osteosclerosis), and
6   extramedullary haemopoiesis.

The white cell and platelet counts may be increased early in the disease but are reduced later. The neutrophil alkaline phosphatase score is frequently raised but may be normal or even low. Red cells may show a defect similar to that seen in paroxysmal nocturnal haemoglobinuria (p. 70) and occasional patients have haemoglobinuria. Hyperuricaemia may

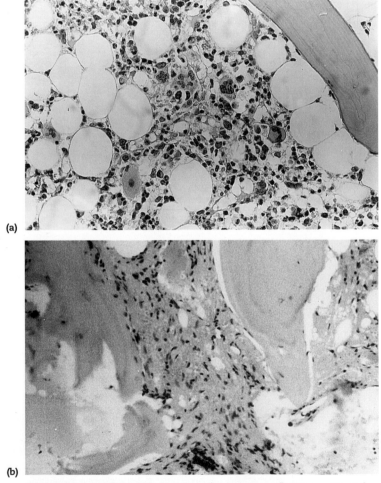

(a)

(b)

Fig. 8.5 Sections of trephine biopsies of bone marrow (haematoxylin and eosin). (a) Specimen from haematologically normal individual. (b) Specimen from a patient with idiopathic myelofibrosis showing replacement of many of the haemopoietic cells by fibroblasts and collagen.

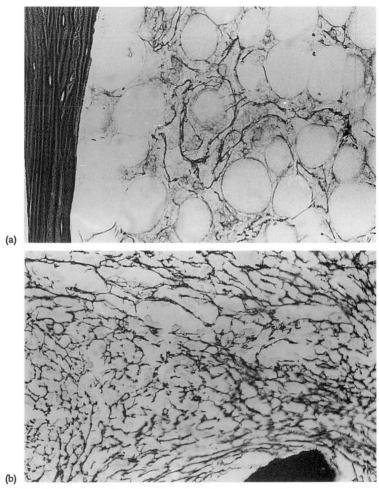

(a)

(b)

Fig. 8.6 Sections of trephine biopsies of bone marrow (silver impregnation of reticulin). (a) Specimen from haematologically normal individual. (b) Specimen from a patient with idiopathic myelofibrosis showing an increase in the quantity of reticulin fibres.

cause gout. X-rays of the axial skeleton show increased bone density (due to osteosclerosis) in about half of the patients.

Marrow aspiration is often unsuccessful and the diagnosis is made by performing a trephine biopsy of the marrow (Figs 8.5 & 8.6, Plates 38, 39). During the early phases of the disease there is hypercellularity of all cell lines in the marrow, including megakaryocytes, and minimal fibrosis. Eventually, there is a marked reduction of haemopoietic tissue associated with a gross increase in reticulin fibres. There is also an increase in

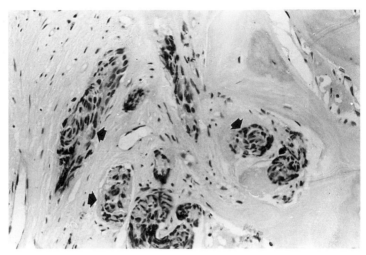

Fig. 8.7 Trephine biopsy of bone marrow showing metastases from a carcinoma (arrows) and fibrosis of the surrounding marrow (i.e. secondary myelofibrosis).

collagen fibres and fibroblasts. A number of diseases such as carcinomatosis, Hodgkin's disease and tuberculosis are sometimes associated with extensive fibrosis of the marrow (Bain & Wickramasinghe 1986) and such causes of secondary myelofibrosis must be excluded (Fig. 8.7).

No treatment is usually given until fairly late in the course of the disease. Markedly anaemic patients require regular blood transfusion. Folic acid, 5 mg daily, is often prescribed as the increased proliferative activity in the marrow increases folate requirements and may cause folate deficiency. Busulphan or hydroxyurea (both carefully administered in low dosage) or low-dose local radiotherapy may be effective in reducing the size of a large spleen that is causing substantial discomfort; allopurinol should be given simultaneously to prevent urate nephropathy and gout. Splenectomy may decrease excessive transfusion requirements or improve troublesome thrombocytopenia when these are related to pooling of cells within the spleen and to hypersplenism. However, there is a significant mortality (10%) from haemorrhage and infection during the post-operative period.

The median survival from diagnosis is 4–5 years. However, survival for 10–20 years is reasonably common. Patients die from bleeding, cardiac failure, infection or thrombosis. Acute leukaemia develops terminally in 10–20% of cases.

References

Bain B.J., Wickramasinghe S.N. (1986) Pathology of the marrow: general considerations. In: Wickramasinghe S.N. *Blood and Bone Marrow, Systemic Pathology*, 3rd edn, Vol 2, p. 73. Churchill Livingstone, Edinburgh.

Hasselbach H.C. (1993) Idiopathic myelofibrosis—an update with particular reference to clinical aspects and prognosis. *Int. J. Clin. Lab. Res.* **23**, 124–138.

Landaw S.A. (1990) Polycythemia vera and other polycythemic states. *Clin. Lab. Med.* **10**, 857–871.

Löfzenberg E., Wahlin A. (1988) Management of polycythaemia vera, essential thrombocythaemia and myelofibrosis with hydroxyurea. *Eur. J. Haematol.* **41**, 375–381.

Pearson T.C., Wetherley-Mein G. (1978) Vascular occlusive episodes and venous hematocrit in primary proliferative polycythaemia. *Lancet* **ii**, 1219–1222.

Rosenthal D.S. (1992) Clinical aspects of chronic myeloproliferative diseases. *Am. J. Med. Sci.* **304**, 109–124.

Szur L., Lewis S.M., Goulden A.W.G. (1959) Polycythaemia vera and its treatment with radioactive phosphorus. *Q. J. Med.* **28**, 397–424.

Talpaz M., Kurzrock R., Kantarjian H., O'Brien S., Gutterman J.U. (1989) Recombinant interferon-alpha therapy of Philadelphia chromosome negative myeloproliferative disorders with thrombocytosis. *Am. J. Med.* **86**, 554–558.

Tefferi A., Hoagland H.C. (1994) Issues in the diagnosis and management of essential thrombocythemia. *Mayo Clin. Proc.* **69**, 651–655.

Tobelem G. (1989) Essential thrombocythaemia. *Clin. Haematol.* **3**, 719–728.

Videbaek A. (1950) Polycythaemia vera. Course and prognosis. *Acta Med. Scand.* **138**, 179–187.

Weinstein I.M. (1991) Idiopathic myelofibrosis: historical review, diagnosis and management. *Blood Rev.* **5**, 98–104.

CHAPTER 9

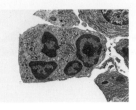

Myelodysplastic Syndromes, Aplastic Anaemia and Pure Red Cell Aplasia

Objectives in learning

1 To understand the concept of the myelodysplastic syndromes.

2 To know the aetiology of acquired aplastic anaemia, including the drugs that have been most commonly reported to cause this syndrome.

3 To know the clinical and laboratory features, the natural history, and the principles of treatment of acquired aplastic anaemia.

4 To understand the difference between aplastic anaemia and pure red cell aplasia.

This chapter deals with two groups of conditions (myelodysplastic syndromes and aplastic anaemias) in which there is bone marrow failure usually due to an abnormality of the haemopoietic stem cells. In the myelodysplastic syndromes the cytopenias are caused by ineffective haemopoiesis; in the aplastic anaemias by a marked insufficiency (aplasia or severe hypoplasia) of haemopoietic tissue. In the third group of conditions discussed, namely pure red cell aplasia, the insufficiency of precursors is confined to the red cell lineage.

Myelodysplastic syndromes

This term is used to describe a group of conditions in which there is evidence of disordered maturation (dysplasia) in one or more of the myeloid cell lineages. Blood-cell production from the dysplastic cell lineages is ineffective and, consequently, may lead to anaemia, thrombocytopenia or neutropenia. The population of dysplastic cells represents an abnormal clone derived from a multipotent myeloid stem cell, that is, the myelodysplastic syndromes are neoplastic disorders. The abnormal clone is stable for a variable period (sometimes for several years). It may, however, generate new clones associated with increasingly ineffective haemopoiesis, or increasing dysfunction of mature cells, or frankly malignant properties. The latter results in the haematological picture of acute myeloid leukaemia. In some patients, the myelodysplastic syndrome is a consequence of previous cytotoxic therapy or irradiation, but in most patients no aetiological factor is readily identifiable. Point mutations affecting the *ras* oncogene (Table 7.5) are found in 20–40% of cases either early or late in the course of the disease. Mutations affecting the *fms* oncogene which codes for the receptor for macrophage colony-stimulating factor (M-CSF) (p. 20) have been found in about 15% of patients.

The majority of patients are elderly. In people over the age of 60 years, the incidence of myelodysplastic syndromes is about 1 in 1500 per year, i.e. six times that of acute myeloid leukaemia (Hamblin & Oscier 1987). Some patients are diagnosed incidentally as a consequence of having a blood count for an unrelated reason. Others present with symptoms referable to anaemia, thrombocytopenia or neutropenia and to functional abnormalities of neutrophils and platelets (i.e. lethargy and dyspnoea, spontaneous bruising and other haemorrhagic symptoms, or infections).

A variety of abnormalities may be seen on the blood film; often only a single abnormality may be found at diagnosis and others appear later. Abnormalities that may be found in the peripheral blood are: macrocytosis of red cells (not due to B_{12} or folate deficiency); a few hypochromic microcytes (when there is sideroblastic erythropoiesis, p. 91); neutrophils with a reduced number of granules (Plate 25) or with the Pelger–Huet phenomenon (bi-lobed spectacle-like nuclei) (Plate 26); and abnormally large platelets. Abnormalities found in the bone marrow include: megaloblastic erythropoiesis (not due to B_{12} or folate deficiency); ring sideroblasts; multinuclearity and irregularities of nuclear outline in erythroblasts; and small megakaryocytes with abnormal nuclei. There may be chromosomal abnormalities such as monosomy 5 or 7, trisomy 8 or partial deletion of the long arm of chromosome 5. The last of these abnormalities is associated with a relatively good prognosis and is found in elderly females with macrocytosis, megakaryocytes containing a single large round nucleus and, sometimes, a high platelet count (5q− syndrome). In contrast to acute myeloid leukaemia, in myelodysplastic syndromes blast cells account for less than 30% of nucleated marrow cells.

On the basis of the haematological findings, the French-American-British (FAB) cooperative group has classified the myelodysplastic syndromes into five categories (Bennett et al. 1982): the details of this classification are shown in Table 9.1. The syndrome of refractory anaemia with ring sideroblasts carries a considerably better prognosis than the others, only a small proportion of cases developing acute leukaemia.

FAB CLASSIFICATION

Syndrome	Peripheral blood	Bone Marrow
Refractory anaemia†	Blasts <1%	Blasts <5%; ring sideroblasts <15%
Refractory anaemia with ring sideroblasts (primary acquired sideroblastic anaemia)	High MCV; dimorphic red-cell picture; blasts <1%	Blasts <5%; ring sideroblasts >15%
RAEB	Blasts <5%	Blasts 5–20%
CMML	Monocyte count >1.0 × 10⁹/l; granulocytes often increased; blasts <5%	Blasts <20%; promonocytes may be increased
RAEB in transformation	Blasts >5% or Auer rods present	Blasts 20–30% or Auer rods present

MCV, mean cell volume; RAEB, refractory anaemia with excess of blasts; CMML, chronic myelomonocytic leukaemia.
† Some patients who have neutropenia and/or thrombocytopenia without anaemia are classified with this category ('refractory cytopenia').
* Beyond the core requirements of medical students but helps the understanding of general concepts.

Table 9.1* FAB classification of myelodysplastic syndromes.

Patients are only treated when symptoms become troublesome. Management of the severe cytopenias is difficult (De Witte 1994) and essentially supportive (e.g. platelet transfusions and appropriate antimicrobial treatment when necessary, regular transfusions of red cells). Drugs that may have some beneficial effect on the blood count include cis-retinoic acid and low doses of cytosine arabinoside. Single-agent chemotherapy with hydroxyurea, etoposide or mercaptopurine may also be of some value. A proportion of cases show a partial response to continuous treatment with granulocyte-macrophage colony-stimulating factor (GM-CSF) and erythropoietin (p. 20). Some young patients with an HLA-matching sibling have been successfully treated with bone marrow transplantation. Once acute myeloid leukaemia develops, most patients die within a few months; the leukaemia responds poorly to chemotherapy.

NON-NEOPLASTIC MYELODYSPLASIA

Dysplastic changes affecting bone marrow cells of one, two or all three haemopoietic lineages are seen in more than 70% of patients with AIDS. This is accompanied by lymphopenia, anaemia, neutropenia and thrombocytopenia in about 40–75% of cases. The peripheral blood cells also show dysplastic changes and these include macrocytosis, left shift of the neutrophils (p. 125), either hypogranularity or abnormally heavy granulation of neutrophils, the acquired Pelger–Huet anomaly (p. 175), binucleate neutrophils and giant neutrophils. The prevalence of cytopenias is much lower in asymptomatic HIV-positive subjects (Center for Disease Control Category II) and increases progressively as the infection progresses. Myelodysplasia occurs even in patients with AIDS who are not receiving myelotoxic drugs. Multiple factors are likely to be involved in its pathogenesis; one such factor may be infection by HIV of bone marrow stromal cells and, possibly, of haemopoietic progenitor cells (Wickramasinghe 1994).

Aplastic anaemia

The causes of aplastic anaemia are summarized in Table 9.2.

ACQUIRED APLASTIC ANAEMIA

Acquired aplastic anaemia is a disorder characterized by pancytopenia, i.e. a reduction in the number of red cells, neutrophils and platelets in the peripheral blood, a marked decrease in the amount of haemopoietic tissue in the bone marrow and the absence of evidence of involvement of the marrow by diseases such as leukaemia, myeloma or carcinoma. It is

CAUSES OF APLASTIC ANAEMIA

Congenital
Fanconi's anaemia

Acquired
Idiopathic
Drugs and chemicals
   Dose-dependent: cytotoxic drugs, benzene
   Idiosyncratic: chloramphenicol, non-steroidal anti-inflammatory drugs
Radiation
Viruses: hepatitis C, Epstein–Barr virus
Paroxysmal nocturnal haemoglobinuria (p. 70)

Table 9.2

an uncommon disease, the prevalence in Europe being between 1 and 3 per 100 000 people.

Aetiology

In about half the cases, no aetiological factors can be identified; such cases are described as having idiopathic acquired aplastic anaemia. In the others, the aplasia is associated with exposure to certain drugs (Malkin et al. 1990) or chemicals, ionizing radiation, or certain viruses.

Most cases of secondary aplastic anaemia result from an idiosyncratic reaction to the use of antirheumatic drugs (e.g. phenylbutazone, indomethacin, ibuprofen or sodium aurothiomalate), chloramphenicol, trimethoprim-sulphamethoxazole (cotrimoxazole) or organic arsenicals. Many other drugs have been less commonly implicated and these include anticonvulsants (phenytoin, carbamazepine), antidiabetic drugs (chlorpropamide and tolbutamide), antithyroid drugs (carbimazole, propylthiouracil), mepacrine and chlorpromazine. Some drugs regularly cause aplastic anaemia if given in sufficiently large doses: these included alkylating agents (e.g. busulphan, melphalan and cyclophosphamide), antipurines, antipyrimidines and antifolates. Benzene is the only industrial chemical which often produces aplastic anaemia if inhaled in sufficient dose; kerosene, carbon tetrachloride and certain insecticides such as DDT and chlordane can also cause aplasia of the marrow.

Aplastic anaemia may develop after a single massive dose of whole body irradiation (e.g. during atomic bomb explosions or radiation accidents). It was also seen in the past following repeated radiotherapy to the spine in patients with ankylosing spondylitis.

Severe aplastic anaemia, usually with a poor prognosis, may rarely develop in children and young adults about 10 weeks after an episode of acute non-A, non-B hepatitis (hepatitis C). Marrow aplasia is also a rare complication of Epstein–Barr virus infection and in this situation may be due to activation of suppressor T cells. In the immunosuppressed recipient of a bone marrow transplant, cytomegalovirus (CMV) infection is sometimes followed by a second phase of marrow failure; the virus infects bone marrow stromal cells and the aplasia may be due to stromal cell damage.

The T-lymphocytes of some patients with acquired aplastic anaemia inhibit the in vitro growth of haemopoietic colonies from autologous and allogeneic bone marrow. This finding, together with the response of about 50% of patients to antilymphocyte globulin, raises the possibility that autoimmune mechanisms may be involved in the aetiology of the aplasia in a number of cases (Bjorkholm 1992).

Pathophysiology

The pancytopenia and marrow aplasia may be the consequence of:

1   damage to the multipotent haemopoietic stem cells which impairs their self-renewal (p. 14) and causes stem cell depletion (e.g. busulphan-related aplasia);

2   damage to the early progenitor cells derived from stem cells (e.g. immunologically mediated damage, some drugs, some viruses) or, rarely,

3   damage to stromal cells (p. 20).

Clinical features

Both idiopathic and secondary aplastic anaemia occur at all ages. The onset is often insidious but may be acute. Symptoms include:

1   lassitude, weakness and shortness of breath due to the anaemia;

2   haemorrhagic manifestations resulting from the thrombocytopenia, and

3   fever and recurrent infections as a consequence of the neutropenia. Haemorrhagic manifestations include epistaxis, bleeding from the gums, menorrhagia, bleeding into the gastrointestinal and urinary tracts and ecchymoses and petechiae. The severity of the symptoms is variable and depends on the severity of the cytopenias. In patients with severe neutropenia and thrombocytopenia, fulminating infections (e.g. pneumonia) and cerebral haemorrhage are common causes of death. In secondary aplastic anaemia, symptoms may appear several weeks or months, or occasionally, one or more years after discontinuation of exposure to the causative drug or chemical. Splenomegaly is rare in aplastic anaemia, and if the spleen is palpable alternative diagnoses should be explored.

Haematological findings

There is a normochromic or macrocytic anaemia, associated with a low absolute reticulocyte count. The platelet count is often below $100 \times 10^9/l$ and may be much lower. A neutropenia and monocytopenia are usually found at some stage of the disease. Some patients also have a reduced absolute lymphocyte count. There is a marked increase in serum and urinary erythropoietin levels.

Markedly hypocellular marrow fragments are usually found in marrow smears, most of the volume of the marrow fragments being made up of fat cells (Plate 13). Haemopoietic cells of all types, including megakaryocytes, are decreased or absent, and in severe aplastic anaemia the majority of the cells seen are plasma cells, lymphocytes and macrophages. Residual erythropoietic cells are morphologically abnormal.

Although the marrow is generally hypocellular, it contains some foci of normal or even increased cellularity. Thus, even in patients with severe aplastic anaemia, marrow aspiration may occasionally yield normocellular or hypercellular fragments. In order to obtain a reliable estimate of marrow cellularity, it is essential to examine histological sections of a trephine biopsy of the iliac crest (Plate 14). This not only provides a larger volume of marrow for study than a single marrow aspirate but also permits the detection of foci of leukaemia cells, myeloma cells or carcinoma cells, if present.

Some patients with acquired aplastic anaemia develop the red cell defect seen in paroxysmal nocturnal haemoglobinuria (p. 70), without or with haemoglobinuria. Occasional patients develop a terminal acute leukaemia.

Diagnosis

Other causes of pancytopenia (particularly, aleukaemic leukaemia) should be considered and excluded before a diagnosis of aplastic anaemia is made. The causes of pancytopenia are summarized in Table 9.3.

Prognosis

Patients with both idiopathic and secondary acquired aplastic anaemia show a highly variable clinical course. About 15% of patients have a

---

CAUSES OF PANCYTOPENIA

Mainly due to a failure of production of cells
Bone marrow infiltration: leukaemia (including aleukaemic leukaemia, p. 145), myeloma, carcinoma (Plate 40), myelofibrosis, lipid storage disorders, marble bone disease
Severe vitamin B_{12} or folate deficiency
Myelodysplastic syndromes
HIV infection
Aplastic or hypoplastic anaemia

Mainly due to an increased peripheral destruction of cells
Splenomegaly
Overwhelming infection
Systemic lupus erythematosus
Paroxysmal nocturnal haemoglobinuria (p. 70)*

* In some cases, there is also an impaired production of cells due to hypoplasia of the marrow.

Table 9.3

severe illness from the outset and die within 3 months of diagnosis. Overall, as many as 50% of cases die within 15 months of diagnosis and 70% within 5 years. Only about 10% make a complete haematological recovery. If a patient survives for longer than 18 months, there is a reasonable chance of prolonged survival and complete recovery. Poor prognostic features include a platelet count less than $20 \times 10^9/l$, a neutrophil count below $0.2 \times 10^9/l$, a reticulocyte count under $10 \times 10^9/l$ and marked hypocellularity of the marrow.

Treatment

If a causative drug or chemical is identified, exposure to this agent should be immediately stopped. Supportive therapy including red-cell transfusions and antibiotics should be administered when necessary; the extent of supportive therapy required depends on the degree of cytopenia. Platelet transfusions are only indicated if haemorrhage becomes a serious problem, as repeated platelet transfusions lead to alloimmunization and a reduction of the efficacy of subsequent platelet transfusions. If marrow transplantation is planned, the administration of blood products should be limited to the bare minimum, since multiple transfusions have an adverse effect on the outcome of transplantation.

Bone marrow transplantation is indicated at diagnosis for patients under 40 years with severe aplastic anaemia (i.e. showing the poor prognostic features mentioned above), particularly if an HLA-compatible sibling donor is available. Long-term survival is seen in 60–80% of cases; graft rejection is more of a problem in aplastic anaemia than in other conditions. Patients who are not transplanted may benefit from treatment with antithymocyte globulin, cyclosporin A, androgens or the anabolic steroid oxymetholone (which causes less virilization of females than androgens).

Fanconi's anaemia

The features of this rare disorder are (Alter 1993):

1 inheritance as an autosomal recessive character;

2 onset of pancytopenia between the ages of 5 and 10 years;

3 frequent association with other congenital abnormalities (e.g. skin pigmentation, short stature, microcephaly, skeletal defects, genital hypoplasia and renal abnormalities);

4 various chromosomal abnormalities (breaks, rearrangements, exchanges and endoreduplications) in cultured lymphocytes and skin fibroblasts;

5 increased number of chromosome breaks per cell after culture with alkylating agents, and

Continued on p. 182

6   increased incidence of acute leukaemia and solid tumours.
There is usually some response to treatment with androgens and corticosteroids. Allogeneic bone marrow transplantation may cure the aplastic
anaemia but does not prevent the appearance of solid tumours.

Pure red cell aplasia

Rarely, aplasia or severe hypoplasia affects only the erythropoietic cells.
Patients with this abnormality have anaemia and reticulocytopenia together with normal white cell and platelet counts. Pure red cell aplasia
may present as an acute self-limiting condition (e.g. when if follows a
parvovirus infection) or as a chronic disorder. The causes of pure red cell
aplasia are listed in Table 9.4.

CAUSES OF PURE RED CELL APLASIA

Congenital
Diamond–Blackfan syndrome (congenital erythroblastopenia or
erythrogenesis imperfecta)

Acquired
Idiopathic
Viral infections: parvovirus B19 (p. 43), Epstein–Barr virus, hepatitis
Drugs: phenytoin sodium, azathioprine
Thymic tumours
Lymphoid malignancies: chronic lymphocytic leukaemia, lymphoma
Other malignant diseases: carcinoma of the bronchus, breast, stomach
   and thyroid
Autoimmune disorders: SLE, rheumatoid arthritis

SLE, systemic lupus erythematosus.

Table 9.4

The parvovirus B19 enters erythroid progenitor cells (by binding to the
P blood group antigen), replicates within these cells and damages them.
In most patients the infection and erythroblastopenia are transient
but in patients with certain congenital or acquired immunological
disorders, there is persistence of the infection and of the red cell
aplasia.
   Immunological mechanisms, both cellular and humoral, may underlie
the aplasia in some patients with pure red cell aplasia (e.g. those with
Continued

thymoma, chronic lymphocytic leukaemia or autoimmune disorders) (Nidorf & Saleem 1990).

Some patients respond to immunosuppressive drugs such as corticosteroids, azathioprine, cyclophosphamide, cyclosporin A or antithymocyte globulin. Patients with persistent parvovirus infection respond to intravenous injections of immunoglobulin.

References

Alter B.P. (1993) Fanconi's anaemia and its variability. *Br. J. Haematol.* **85**, 9–14.
Bennett J.M., Catovsky D., Daniel M.T., Flandrin G., Galton D.A.G., Gralnick H.R., Sultan C. (1982) Proposals for the classification of the myelodysplastic syndromes. *Br. J. Haematol.* **51**, 189–199.
Bjorkholm M. (1992) Aplastic anaemia: pathogenetic mechanisms and treatment with special reference to immunomodulation. *J. Int. Med.* **231**, 575–582.
De Witte T. (1994) New treatment approaches for myelodysplastic syndrome and secondary leukaemias. *Ann. Oncol.* **5**, 401–408.
Hamblin T.J., Oscier D.G. (1987) The myelodysplastic syndrome – a practical guide. *Hematol. Oncol.* **5**, 19–34.
Malkin D., Koren G., Saunders E.F. (1990) Drug-induced aplastic anaemia: pathogenesis and clinical aspects. *Am. J. Pediatr. Hematol. Oncol.* **12**, 402–410.
Nidorf D., Saleem A. (1990) Immunosuppressive mechanisms in pure red cell aplasia—a review. *Ann. Clin. Lab. Sci.* **20**, 214–219.
Wickramasinghe S.N. (1994) Bone marrow damage in AIDS. In: Bhatt H.R., James V.H.T., Besser G.M., Bottazzo G.F., Keen H. (eds.) *Advances in Thomas Addison's Diseases*, Vol 2, pp. 339–355. Journal of Endocrinology Ltd, Bristol.

Reviews

Camitta B.M., Storb R., Thomas E.D. (1982) Aplastic anaemia. *N. Eng. J. Med.* **306**, 645 & 712.
Dessypris E.N. (1991) The biology of pure red cell aplasia. *Semin. Hematol.* **28**, 275–284.
Gordon-Smith E.C. (ed.) (1989) Aplastic anaemia. *Clin. Haematol.* **2**, 1–190.
Gordon-Smith E.C., Issaragrisil S. (1992) Epidemiology of aplastic anaemia. Baillière's Clinical Haematology, International Practice and Research, Vol 5/No 2, pp. 475–491.
Keoffler H.P. (ed.) (1992) Myelodysplastic syndromes. *Hematol./Oncol. Clin. N. Am.* **6**, 485–728.
Shahidi N.T. (1990) *Aplastic Anemia and Other Bone Marrow Failure Syndromes.* Springer–Verlag, Berlin.

CHAPTER 10

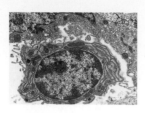

Myeloma, other Paraproteinaemias and Lymphoma

Objectives in learning

1 To understand the meaning of the term paraprotein and to know the various clinical situations in which a paraprotein may be found.

2 To have a moderately detailed knowledge of the pathology, clinical features and diagnosis of myelomatosis and to understand the principles of treatment of this disorder.

3 To understand the pathological and clinical features and the principles of treatment of Hodgkin's disease and the non-Hodgkin's lymphomas. Details of the various histological classifications of non-Hodgkin's lymphomas need not be known.

Multiple myeloma

Multiple myeloma is a disease arising from the malignant transformation of a B cell or, possibly, a pre-B or earlier cell (Barlogie *et al.* 1989; Jensen *et al.* 1991). The differentiating cells of the malignant clone have the morphology of plasma cells or plasmacytoid lymphocytes, have clonally rearranged immunoglobulin genes and usually secrete a monoclonal immunoglobulin (Ig), a monoclonal light chain, or both. Such monoclonal proteins are called paraproteins; they consist of structurally identical molecules and, therefore, produce a discrete band (M band) on electrophoresis. The primary site of proliferation of the malignant cells is the bone marrow which shows many nodules of tumour tissue as well as diffuse interstitial infiltration (Fig. 10.1). Osteoclasts are stimulated by IL-6 secreted by cells in the vicinity of the myeloma cells and this, together with the expansion of the tumour cell mass, leads to multiple well-defined osteolytic lesions, radiological changes resembling those of generalized osteoporosis, and hypercalcaemia. Marrow infiltration also causes impairment of haemopoiesis and haematological abnormalities. Some patients with IgA paraproteins (which tend to polymerize) and a few patients with high levels of IgG3 paraproteins have a substantially raised plasma viscosity and may suffer from the hyperviscosity syndrome (p. 186). Light chains are filtered through the glomeruli and are found in

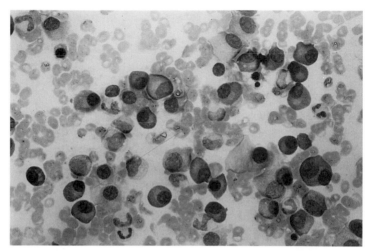

Fig. 10.1 Bone marrow smear from a patient with multiple myeloma showing infiltration by myeloma cells. There are only a few normal haemopoietic cells.

the urine; they may eventually damage the renal tubules. In 10% of patients, the paraprotein is converted into deposits of amyloid in various tissues. Levels of normal Ig are reduced and in advanced disease there is a reduction in circulating T cells. Extramedullary tumour deposits develop frequently.

CLINICAL FEATURES

The incidence of myeloma is 3–6 cases per 100 000 of the population per year. Most patients are between the ages of 50 and 70 years. There is a prolonged asymptomatic phase which may last for a number of years. The most common presenting symptom is bone pain usually over the lumbar spine. Pathological fractures are frequent and often affect the lower thoracic and upper lumbar vertebrae and the ribs. Compression fractures of the vertebrae may damage the spinal cord or spinal roots and cause neurological symptoms. Large tumours may form in relation to any bone and cause pressure symptoms.

Renal failure may be found at presentation or develop during the course of the disease. Chronic renal failure commonly results from obstruction of renal tubules by proteinaceous casts leading to tubular atrophy and interstitial fibrosis (myeloma kidney). Renal dysfunction may also result from the toxic effects of light chains on tubule cells, the deposition of light chains in glomeruli and amyloidosis. Acute renal failure may be precipitated by dehydration, or caused by hypercalcaemia or hyperuricaemia.

Other features of myelomatosis include:

1   symptoms of anaemia (p. 26);

2   recurrent bacterial infections due mainly to decreased levels of normal Ig but also to neutropenia;

3   systemic symptoms of hypercalcaemia such as anorexia, vomiting, lethargy, stupor or coma, and

4   peripheral and autonomic neuropathy, macroglossia, cardiomegaly, diarrhoea and carpal tunnel syndrome due to amyloidosis.

Peripheral neuropathy may also be caused by infiltration of nerves by plasma cells or by a direct toxic effect of the paraprotein. The hyperviscosity syndrome may occasionally develop. This is characterized by neurological disturbances (dizziness, somnolence and coma), cardiac failure and haemorrhagic manifestations. Spontaneous haemorrhages may also occur in the absence of hyperviscosity due to an adverse effect of the paraprotein on coagulation and platelet function and, in the later stages of the disease, due to thrombocytopenia. A few paraproteins are cryoglobulins and may cause symptoms such as urticaria and acrocyanosis, when the patient becomes cold.

LABORATORY FINDINGS

A normochromic normocytic anaemia is common. When the disease is advanced, thrombocytopenia and neutropenia may also be found. The blood film may show a leucoerythroblastic picture and occasional plasma cells; red cells may show an increased tendency to form rouleaux (Plate 47) and the paraprotein may cause an increased basophilic staining of the background in between red cells. The erythrocyte sedimentation rate (ESR) is often raised, sometimes to more than 100 mm/h. The serum uric acid is raised in about half the cases (and may contribute to the renal damage).

Bone marrow aspirates usually contain a greatly increased proportion of plasma cells (Plates 41, 43). The latter may either appear normal or show various atypical features such as marked pleomorphism, pronounced multinuclearity, immaturity of the nucleus (i.e. finely distributed chromatin and nucleoli and dissociation between nuclear and cytoplasmic maturation). Some aspirates may show only a slight increase in plasma cells (5–10% of nucleated marrow cells as compared with 0.1–2% in normal marrow) and others may show no increase. The latter results from the multifocal nature of the plasma cell infiltrate.

Electrophoresis of serum usually demonstrates the monoclonal Ig as a discrete band (M-band) and the nature of the paraprotein can be determined by immunofixation. Each Ig class may be quantitated using rate immunonephalometry. Light chains (also called Bence-Jones proteins) cannot usually be detected in the serum except when there is impairment of renal function. They are present in urine and are best detected and studied by electrophoresis and immunofixation. Conversely, whole Ig molecules only appear in the urine when there is renal damage. In 50% of patients with myeloma, the paraprotein is IgG, in 25% it is IgA, in 20% it is light chain only and in 1–2% it is IgD or IgE. IgM-producing myelomas are extremely rare. Over half the patients with an IgG- or IgA-secreting myeloma have monoclonal light chains in their urine; in two-thirds of these patients the light chain is $\varkappa$ and in the remainder it is λ. In 1–2% of patients with myeloma, paraprotein cannot be detected in either serum or concentrated urine (non-secretory myeloma).

Serum levels of β_2-microglobulin (the light chain of the HLA class I glycoproteins) correlates with tumour mass.

DIAGNOSIS

This is often based on the finding of at least two of the following three features:

1 a monoclonal Ig in the serum or monoclonal light chains in the urine or both;

2 an increased proportion of plasma cells (often with atypical features) in marrow aspirates, and

3 discrete osteolytic lesions on X-ray studies (Fig. 10.2).

The differential diagnosis is from a benign paraproteinaemia (p. 190).

TREATMENT

Cytotoxic drugs are usually reserved for patients with extensive or symptomatic bone lesions, hypercalcaemia, bone marrow failure, substantial Bence-Jones proteinuria or any renal dysfunction (Samson 1994; MacLennan et al. 1994). Patients over 65 years are usually treated with melphalan or cyclophosphamide given orally with or without prednisolone either intermittently (for 4–5 days every 6 weeks) or, in smaller doses, continuously. Cyclophosphamide may also be given intravenously every week. Most patients respond, with an improvement in symptoms, a rise in haemoglobin (Hb) and a gradual reduction in the paraprotein levels. Treatment reduces the tumour mass and is usually stopped when the paraprotein level stops falling (plateau phase). Combination chemotherapy is more effective in inducing disease regression than single drugs and is recommended in younger patients; it may also be given to patients who fail to respond to single drug therapy. The usual

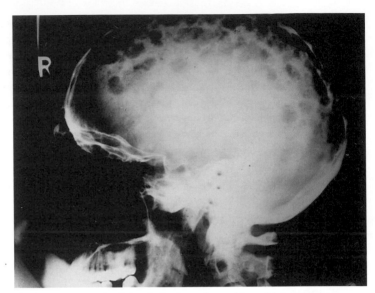

Fig. 10.2 Radiograph of the skull of a patient with multiple myeloma showing multiple discrete radiolucent lesions with no sclerosis at the margin.

drug combinations are (MacLennan et al. 1992; MacLennan et al. 1994; Samson 1994); ABCM (adriamycin, BCNU, cyclophosphamide and melphalan) or VAD (vincristine, adriamycin and dexamethasone) and several cycles of chemotherapy are administered. Some patients who remit have also been treated with a single high dose of melphalan intravenously followed by autologous bone marrow transplantation (p. 159) and this approach results in prolonged complete remissions in a proportion of cases.

A decompression laminectomy is required in cases with impending and established compression paraplegia. Local radiotherapy rapidly relieves bone pain and has an important role in the management of spinal cord compression. Acute hypercalcaemia is treated with rehydration together with prednisolone, mithramycin, calcitonin or biphosphonates.

Current trials indicate that α-interferon may have a beneficial effect when used together with chemotherapy in the remission induction phase and during the plateau phase (Mandelli et al. 1990).

PROGNOSIS

The median survival from diagnosis is 2–3 years. Asymptomatic patients with an Hb greater than 10 g/dl and blood urea less than or equal to

8 mmol/l have a 75% chance of surviving 2 years. By contrast, patients who are restricted in their activity and who have either an Hb less than or equal to 7.5 g/dl or a blood urea greater than 10 mmol/l have only a 10% chance of surviving 2 years. Patients eventually become refractory to chemotherapy and die of renal failure or infection. A few patients develop a myelodysplastic syndrome or terminal acute myeloid leukaemia or immunoblastic lymphoma.

Solitary plasmacytoma

Solitary tumours consisting of malignant plasma cells may be found in the bone marrow or in extramedullary sites such as the upper respiratory tract. It is usual to find a monoclonal Ig in the serum or monoclonal light chains in the urine, or both. In the case of extramedullary plasmacytomas, there is often no evidence of tumour elsewhere and the prognosis after excision followed by local radiotherapy is very good.

Other paraproteinaemias

WALDENSTRÖM'S MACROGLOBULINAEMIA

In this condition, there is a malignant monoclonal proliferation of a cell belonging to the B-lineage. The incidence is about 10% of that of multiple myeloma. The tumour cells are found in peripheral lymphoid tissue, bone marrow and other tissues and, in some patients, also in the peripheral blood. They have the morphology of plasmacytoid lymphocytes and secrete an IgM paraprotein and thus differ from myeloma cells which very rarely secrete this class of paraprotein. Symptoms result both from tissue infiltration and from hyperviscosity of the blood caused by the paraprotein. Unlike in multiple myeloma, osteolytic lesions are rare.

HEAVY CHAIN DISEASES

In these rare paraproteinaemias, the B-lineage-derived malignant clone secretes γ, α or μ heavy chains rather than complete Ig molecules. The clinical picture is that of a lymphoma; α-chain disease is characterized by severe malabsorption due to infiltration of the small intestine by lymphoma cells.

OTHER LYMPHOPROLIFERATIVE DISORDERS

A paraprotein may also be found in chronic cold haemagglutinin disease (p. 69), and in some patients with malignant lymphoma or chronic lymphocytic leukaemia.

BENIGN PARAPROTEINAEMIA (BENIGN MONOCLONAL GAMMOPATHY OR MONOCLONAL GAMMOPATHY OF UNCERTAIN SIGNIFICANCE, MGUS)

A paraprotein is found in the serum in 0.1–1.0% for normal adults and in 3% of subjects over 70 years. A high proportion of such individuals suffer from a condition termed benign paraproteinaemia that does not require treatment; in this condition, the abnormal clone, derived from the B-cell lineage, behaves like a benign neoplasm. Benign paraproteinaemia is characterized by:

1 the absence of osteolytic lesions;

2 the presence of relatively low levels of serum paraprotein ($< 20\,g/l$) which remain stable over a long period of follow-up;

3 the absence of light chains or the presence of very low concentrations ($< 500\,mg/day$) of light chains in the urine;

4 normal levels of Ig's of classes other than the paraprotein class;

5 the finding of less than 5–10% of plasma cells in the bone marrow (i.e. only a slight plasmacytosis in the marrow), and

6 the absence of marrow failure.

Malignant lymphomas

The malignant lymphomas are tumours of lymphoid tissue (e.g. lymph nodes, spleen and mucosa-associated lymphoid tissue). The transformed cell is either a cell of lymph node origin giving rise to Reed–Sternberg cells (see below) in the case of Hodgkin's lymphoma or a cell belonging to the lymphocyte series and not generating Reed–Sternberg cells in the case of non-Hodgkin's lymphomas. The expansion of the malignant cell clone causes a partial or complete loss of normal lymph node architecture and a progressive enlargement of lymph nodes. Although the bone marrow and peripheral blood may contain lymphoma cells at some stage, the predominant pathological manifestations are in extramedullary tissue (usually lymph nodes).

HODGKIN'S DISEASE

In this condition the affected lymph nodes (Fig. 10.3) are infiltrated by abnormal mononucleate cells, large binucleate or multinucleate cells called Reed–Sternberg cells, lymphocytes, plasma cells, macrophages, eosinophils and fibrous tissue. The Reed–Sternberg cells and their mononuclear counterparts possess vesicular nuclei with prominent eosinophilic nucleoli (Plate 42). They are the malignant cells but their origin is still controversial; at least in some patients they may be derived from an early lymphoid cell. The other cell types infiltrating the lymph

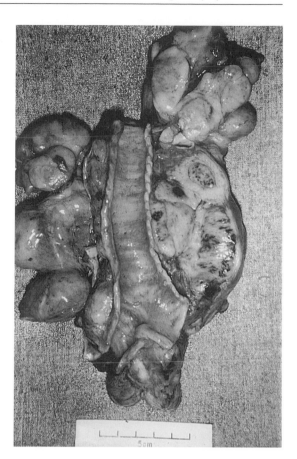

Fig. 10.3 Post-mortem findings in a patient with advanced Hodgkin's disease. The mediastinal glands are greatly enlarged due to infiltration by tumour tissue.

nodes are probably normal cells that are reacting against the tumour cells. The affected lymph nodes of 40–50% of patients contain the Epstein–Barr (EB) virus genome in the Reed–Sternberg cells suggesting that in these cases the EB virus may be involved in the development of Hodgkin's disease.

Clinical features

The age-related incidence curves are bimodal with one peak in young adults and the other in old age. The male:female ratio is about 2:1, but the nodular sclerosing type of the disease (p. 193) is predominantly seen in young females. The disease has an insidious onset. The most common presentation is gradual enlargement of one group of lymph nodes. The disease then spreads to adjacent lymph node areas via the lymphatics and eventually metastasizes via the blood to extranodal sites. The cervical lymph nodes are affected first in 55% of cases and the mediastinal, axillary, abdominal and inguinal glands in 15, 10, 5 and 9%, respectively (Selby & McElwain 1987). The enlarged glands vary in size from 1 to 8 cm in diameter and are usually discrete, painless and rubbery. Splenomegaly may be present (Fig. 10.4). Hepatomegaly and involvement of other extra-nodal tissue is usually seen late in the course of the disease; the affected tissues may include the skin, stomach, small intestine, bone, lung and central nervous system.

Systemic symptoms are frequently present and may sometimes precede the detection of lymphadenopathy. Such symptoms include fever, pruritus, weight loss, lassitude, night sweats. Sometimes the fever is cyclic with several days of high swinging fever alternating with afebrile periods (Pel–Ebstein fever).

Haematological features

There is usually a normochromic normocytic anaemia and a high ESR. A neutrophil leucocytosis is seen in 30% of patients and eosinophilia in some cases. Marrow infiltration may occur and lead to a leucoerythroblastic blood picture. Lymphopenia due to a reduction in T-lymphocytes occurs late in the disease and is associated with an impairment of cell-mediated immunity and a consequent susceptibility to certain viral, fungal and protozoal infections and tuberculosis.

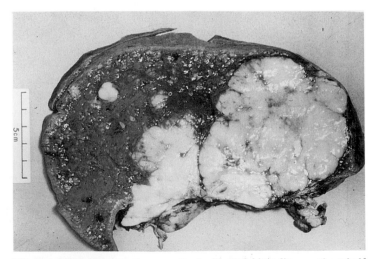

Fig. 10.4 Enlarged spleen from a patient with Hodgkin's disease. About half the cut surface of the spleen is occupied by masses of pale lymphoma tissue.

RYE CLASSIFICATION

Subgroup	Characteristics	Cases (%)	Surviving 5 years (%)
Lymphocyte predominance	Infiltrate consists largely of small lymphocytes. There are only a few eosinophils, Reed–Sternberg cells and mononuclear Hodgkin's cells	15	70
Nodular sclerosing	The node is divided by broad bands of connective tissue into nodules containing a mixture of Reed–Sternberg cells, mononuclear Hodgkin's cells, lymphocytes, plasma cells, macrophages and eosinophils	40	60
Mixed cellularity	There are no broad bands of connective tissue. The node is diffusely infiltrated with the same mixture of cell types as above. Reed–Sternberg cells are readily seen. Fibrosis and focal necrosis are common	30	30
Lymphocyte depletion	Mononuclear Hodgkin's cells and Reed–Sternberg cells are present in large numbers. Relatively few lymphocytes are seen and there may be diffuse fibrosis	15	20

Table 10.1 Rye classification of the histological appearances of lymph nodes in Hodgkin's disease.

Histopathology of lymph nodes

There is complete or partial loss of the normal architecture due to infiltration by malignant and inflammatory cells. The diagnosis is based on finding Reed–Sternberg cells in the appropriate cellular background of mononuclear Hodgkin's cells, lymphocytes, neutrophil polymorphs, eosinophils and plasma cells (Kaplan 1980). Four different histopathological appearances are encountered in Hodgkin's disease and these are described in Table 10.1.

Staging and treatment

The extent of dissemination of malignant cells at presentation influences both the prognosis and the choice of therapy. Clinical staging involves not only a full clinical examination but also various investigations including chest X-ray, trephine biopsy of the bone marrow, and computed tomography (CT) scanning of the abdomen. Table 10.2 summarizes the features of the Ann Arbor staging system which is commonly used to assess the spread of the disease. Each stage is subdivided into A or B depending on whether systemic symptoms are absent or present, respectively. If a staging laparotomy with splenectomy, a wedge-biopsy of the liver and abdominal lymph node biopsy are performed, about one-third of cases initially considered to be in stages I or II are also found to have subdiaphragmatic disease and have to be placed in stages III or IV. However, most clinicians do not regularly perform staging laparotomies in such cases as the improved accuracy in staging achieved in this way is not reflected in improved survival. This is mainly because patients who relapse after radiotherapy respond well to chemotherapy.

Megavoltage radiotherapy is the treatment of choice for stages I and IIA, cyclical combination chemotherapy or radiotherapy for stage IIB and cyclical combination chemotherapy for stages III and IV and for patients who relapse after radiotherapy. Chemotherapy is sometimes also used as first line therapy for stage IIA with involvement of three or more nodal sites. Radiotherapy may be used following chemotherapy for the treatment of bulky or painful nodal or extranodal tumour masses and ulcerating skin lesions. The most commonly used drug combinations are mustine, vincristine (Oncovin), procarbazine and prednisolone (MOPP) or adriamycin, bleomycin, vinblastine and dacarbazine (ABVD) or vari-

ANN ARBOR STAGING	
Stage	**Characteristics**
I	Involvement of one lymph node area
II	Involvement of two or more lymph node areas on the same side of the diaphragm
III	Involvement of lymph nodes on both sides of the diaphragm with or without involvement of the spleen
IV	Involvement of one or more extranodal sites (e.g. liver, marrow, lung)

Table 10.2 Basic features of the Ann Arbor staging system.

ations of these regimes. Usually six cycles of chemotherapy are given. One form of treatment used in relapsed cases (Bonadonna & Santoro 1990; Goldstone & Linch 1992) is intensive chemotherapy or radiation therapy followed by autologous bone marrow transplantation (p. 159). This approach offers a 50% chance of a 3–5-year survival.

Patients treated with alkylating agents show an increased incidence of myelodysplastic syndromes and acute myeloid leukaemia and to a lesser extent of non-Hodgkin's lymphoma or carcinoma.

Prognosis

This is related to both the histological type and clinical staging. Radiotherapy cures (10-year disease-free survival) over 90% of patients in stage I and over 80% in stage II. Combination chemotherapy induces a complete remission in 80% of cases in stages IIIB and IV and a 5-year disease-free survival in 50%.

NON-HODGKIN'S LYMPHOMA

A number of biologically distinct tumours arising from cells of lymphoid tissue are included in this category. Studies using monoclonal antibodies known to react with cell surface antigens present at various stages of normal lymphopoiesis (p. 21) have indicated that about 75% of non-Hodgkin's lymphomas (including all follicular lymphomas) arise from cells of the B-cell lineage and most of the remainder from those of the T-cell lineage. The cluster differentiation (CD) antigens useful in diagnosing B-cell lymphomas include CD19, CD20 and CD22, and those useful in diagnosing T-cell lymphomas include CD2, CD3, CD4, CD7 and CD8. The clonality of these tumours has been established by the demonstration of clonal heavy and light chain gene rearrangements in B-cell lymphomas and clonal T-cell receptor gene rearrangements in T-cell lymphomas. The non-Hodgkin's lymphomas are currently classified into a number of types largely on the basis of the histological and cytological features of the tumour tissue (Rappaport 1977; Lennert 1981; Swerdlow 1992). On the basis of clinicopathological correlations, these various types are assigned one of two or three grades of malignancy (low-grade and high-grade, or low-grade, intermediate-grade and high-grade).

Aetiology

The aetiology is unknown. Patients with certain inherited or acquired immune deficiency syndromes (e.g. sex-linked agammaglobulinaemia, AIDS, patients with renal and heart transplants receiving immunosuppressive therapy) have an increased incidence of non-Hodgkin's lymphoma, as do survivors of the atomic bomb explosions in Japan. The tumours in immunodeficient individuals are often associated with EB virus. Lymphomas developing post-transplantation may be preceded by an EB-virus-related polyclonal lymphoproliferative disorder. The African type of Burkitt's lymphoma is associated with malaria, EB virus infection (Bird & Britton 1982) and one of three specific chromosome translocations which result in the activation of an oncogene, myc (p. 140). In most cases of follicular lymphoma, a chromosomal translocation, t(14;18), juxtaposes the bcl-2 oncogene on chromosome 18 next to the heavy chain locus on chromosome 14 (p. 140).

Clinical features

Painless enlargement of lymph nodes is the most frequent complaint. In general, the extent of spread of the disease at presentation is greater than in Hodgkin's disease. Hepatosplenomegaly is often found and other extranodal sites such as the bone marrow, nervous system, nasopharynx, gastrointestinal tract and skin are commonly involved. Constitutional symptoms are less frequent than in Hodgkin's disease and occur late in the course of the illness.

Haematological features

A normochromic normocytic anaemia is usually found and may be due to marrow infiltration, autoimmune haemolysis or splenomegaly and hypersplenism. Lymphoma cells may be present in the blood, with or without an associated lymphocytosis. In about 10% of patients there is an IgG or IgM paraprotein.

Histopathology of lymph nodes

Rappaport (1977) divided non-Hodgkin's lymphomas into nodular (follicular) or diffuse, depending on whether the tumour cells formed discrete nodules or diffusely infiltrated the lymph nodes (Figs 10.5 & 10.6). The tumours were then subclassified, according to the cell types present, into well or poorly differentiated lymphocytic lymphomas, histiocytic lymphomas, mixed lymphocytic and histiocytic lymphomas and undifferentiated lymphomas. This classification has been replaced by newer ones largely because surface marker studies of tumour cells have shown that in most tumours, cells described by Rappaport as histiocytes are in fact not histiocytes but lymphoid cells.

One of several schemes now used for the histopathological categorization of non-Hodgkin's lymphomas is the Kiel classification. This is based on the hypothesis that such tumours are derived from normal counterparts seen during the antigen-stimulated proliferation of B or T cells in peripheral lymphoid tissue and that the malignant cells retain

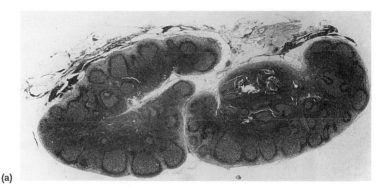

(a)

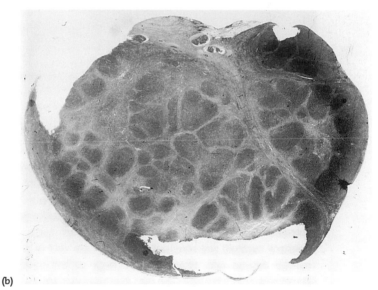

(b)

Fig. 10.5 (a) Section of antigen-stimulated human lymph node. The lymphoid follicles are confined to the cortex (B-cell area) and have an outer darkly-staining zone containing small lymphocytes and a pale germinal centre containing centroblasts (follicle centre cells), dendritic cells and macrophages. (b) Section of a lymph node infiltrated by a follicular (nodular) lymphoma. Note that the nodules of lymphoma cells are found throughout the lymph node, being present not only in the cortex but also in the paracortex (normally a T-cell area) and medulla (normally a follicle-free T- and B-cell area). (Courtesy of Dr R.D. Goldin.)

Fig. 10.6 Section of lymph node affected by a diffuse lymphoma. The diffuse infiltration by lymphoma cells has resulted in a complete loss of nodal architecture. (Courtesy of Dr R.D. Goldin.)

morphological similarity with their putative normal counterparts, being unable to mature further. The cytological stages through which B cells progress following stimulation with specific antigen include centrocytes (which are small or large cells with cleaved nuclei), lymphoblasts (which are medium sized cells with rounded nuclei and inconspicuous nucleoli), centroblasts (which are large cells with rounded nuclei and several peripheral nucleoli) and immunoblasts (which are very large cells with a rounded nucleus and, often, a single large central nucleolus). Both centrocytes and centroblasts are seen in normal germinal centres and the end-result of antigen-mediated stimulation of B cells is the formation of plasma cells or memory B cells. The features of the Kiel classification are given in Table 10.3.

Treatment and prognosis

The staging system described for Hodgkin's disease is used to determine the extent of dissemination at presentation; however, the clinical stage correlates less well with prognosis than in Hodgkin's disease. Patients with low-grade tumours are often in stage IV at presentation and an appreciable percentage of patients with high-grade tumours are in stages I or II.

Some asymptomatic patients with low-grade tumours in whom the disease progresses very slowly need not be treated at presentation.

KIEL CLASSIFICATION

Low-grade malignancy
Lymphocytic (B, T)
Lymphoplasmacytic (B)
Centrocytic (B)
Centrocytic/centroblastic (B)

High-grade malignancy
Centroblastic (B)
Lymphoblastic (B, T)
  Burkitt type
  convoluted-cell type
  others
Immunoblastic (B, T)

Table 10.3 Kiel classification of non-Hodgkin's lymphoma.

Symptomatic patients or patients with progressive disease may be treated with local radiotherapy if in stages I and II or with chemotherapy if in stages III and IV. Either single agent therapy with chlorambucil or combination chemotherapy with cyclophosphamide, vincristine (Oncovin) and prednisolone (COP) are effective. Although most patients with low-grade lymphomas are incurable, their median survival is relatively long, being about 7 years.

In patients with high-grade lymphomas, radiotherapy is used for stage I disease and combination chemotherapy for stages II–IV. Radiotherapy cures many patients in stage I. Intensive chemotherapy induces complete remissions in about half the patients and cures about 20–30%. A variety of combinations of cytotoxic drugs are being used; one well-tried combination is cyclophosphamide, hydroxydaunorubicin (adriamycin), vincristine (Oncovin) and prednisolone (CHOP). High-dose chemotherapy or radiation therapy followed by autologous or allogeneic bone marrow transplantation (p. 158) can cure some relapsed patients (Goldstone & Linch 1992).

SOME VARIETIES OF NON-HODGKIN'S LYMPHOMA

Burkitt's lymphoma is a B-lymphoblastic lymphoma with specific cytological and histological features. Affected African children commonly present with a jaw tumour and non-African patients with an abdominal tumour.

The Sézary syndrome and mycosis fungoides are cutaneous T-cell lymphomas. Sézary's syndrome is characterized by itchy erythroderma, exfoliative dermatitis, lymphadenopathy, hepatosplenomegaly and the presence of some lymphoma cells with cerebriform nuclei (Sézary cells) in the peripheral blood. Mycosis fungoides is characterized by the

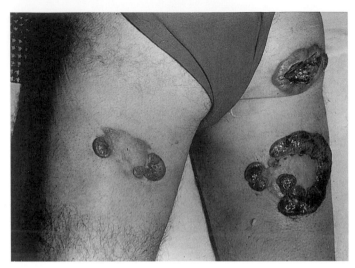

Fig. 10.7 Skin lesions in a patient with mycosis fungoides (a cutaneous T-cell lymphoma). The name of the disease is misleading: this condition is not caused by a fungus.

formation of plaques and nodules of tumour cells in the skin (Fig. 10.7). In this condition, extracutaneous spread only occurs late in the course of the disease.

Adult T-cell leukaemia/lymphoma

This is a condition that develops in some carriers of the HTLV-1 retrovirus; the virus is clonally integrated into the DNA of the malignant cell but the site of integration may vary from case to case. The disease is most common in Japan, the West Indies and South America and in immigrants from these areas, but has also been found sporadically in several other countries. The malignant cells belong to the T-cell lineage, are pleomorphic and often have multilobed or convoluted nuclei; they are found in the lymph nodes and in some cases also in the blood and bone marrow. Common clinical features are skin infiltration, lymphadenopathy and bone lesions. There is a poor prognosis and a poor response to chemotherapy.

References

Barlogie B., Epstein J., Selvanayagam P., Alexanian R. (1989) Plasma cell myeloma—new biological insights and advances in therapy. *Blood* **73**, 865–879.

Bird A.G., Britton S. (1982) The relationship between Epstein–Barr virus and lymphoma. *Semin. Haematol.* **19**, 285–300.

Bonadonna G., Santoro A. (1990) Current issues in the management of advanced Hodgkin's disease. *Blood Rev.* **4**, 69–73.

Goldstone A.H., Linch D.C. (1992) Bone marrow transplantation in the malignant lymphomas. In: Hoffbrand A.V. & Brenner M.K. (eds.) *Recent Advances in Haematology*, Vol 6, pp. 149–172. Churchill Livingstone, Edinburgh.

Jensen G.S., Mant M.J., Belch A.J., Berenson J.R., Ruether B.A., Pilarski L.M. (1991) Selective expression of CD45 isoforms defines CALLA+ monoclonal B-lineage cells in peripheral blood from myeloma patients as late stage B cells. *Blood* **78**, 711–719.

Kaplan H.S. (1980) *Hodgkin's disease*, 2nd edn. Harvard University Press, Cambridge, Massachusetts.

Lennert K. (1981) *Malignant lymphomas other than Hodgkin's disease*. Springer–Verlag, New York.

MacLennan I.C.M., Chapman C., Dunn J., Kelly K. (1992) Combined chemotherapy with ABCM versus melphalan for treatment of myelomatosis. *Lancet* **339**, 200–205.

MacLennan I.C.M., Drayson M., Dunn J. (1994) Multiple myeloma. *Br. Med. J.* **308**, 1033–1036.

Mandelli F., Avvisati G., Amadori S., Boccadoro M., Gernone A., Lauta V.M., Marmont F., Petrucci M.T., Tribalto M., Vegna M.L., Dammacco F., Pileri A. (1990) Maintenance treatment with recombinant interferon alpha-2b in patients with multiple myeloma responding to conventional induction chemotherapy. *N. Engl. J. Med.* **322**, 1430–1434.

Rappaport H. (1977) Histological classification: non-Hodgkin's lymphoma. In: Janes S.E. & Grodden T. (eds.) *Cancer Treatment Reports* **61**, 1037–1048.

Samson D. (1994) Multiple myeloma: current treatment. *Postgrad. Med. J.* **70**, 404–410.

Selby P., McElwain T.J. (eds.) (1987) *Hodgkin's disease*. Blackwell Scientific Publications, Oxford.

Swerdlow S.H. (1992) *Biopsy Interpretation of Lymph Nodes*. Raven Press, New York.

Reviews

Aisenberg A.C. (1991) *Malignant Lymphoma: Biology, Natural History and Treatment*. Lea & Febiger, Philadelphia.

Armitage J.O. (ed.) (1991) Non-Hodgkin's lymphoma. *Hematol./Oncol. Clin. N. Am.* **5**, 845–1093.

Barlogie B (ed.) (1992) Multiple myeloma. *Hematol./Oncol. Clin. N. Am.* **6**, 211–484.

Collins R.H. (1990) The pathogenesis of Hodgkin's disease. *Blood Rev.* **4**, 61–72.

Jarrett R.F. (1992) Hodgkin's disease. *Clin. Haematol.* **5**, 57–80.

Ramot B., Rechavi G. (1992) Non-Hodgkin's lymphomas and paraproteinaemias. *Clin. Haematol.* **5**, 81–100.

CHAPTER 11

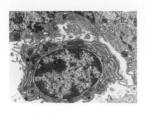

Haemostasis, Abnormal Bleeding and Anticoagulant Therapy

Objectives in learning

1 To know the morphology and function of platelets and the relationship between the concentration of platelets in peripheral blood and the extent of abnormal bleeding.

2 To know about the diseases associated with: (a) a failure of platelet production; and (b) a shortened platelet life-span, especially idiopathic autoimmune thrombocytopenic purpura.

3 To know the main sequence of events in both the intrinsic and extrinsic clotting pathways.

4 To understand normal fibrinolysis and the principles of fibrinolytic therapy.

5 To know the principles underlying tests for the intrinsic system, extrinsic system and final common pathway of blood coagulation, including the prothrombin time, activated partial thromboplastin time and thrombin time.

6 To know the principles of investigation of a patient suspected of having a haemostatic defect.

7 To know the mode of inheritance, clinical presentation, method of diagnosis and principles of treatment of haemophilia, factor IX deficiency and von Willebrand's disease.

8 To know the effects of vitamin K deficiency and liver disease on the clotting mechanisms.

9 To know the alterations in the haemostatic and fibrinolytic mechanisms associated with disseminated intravascular coagulation (DIC) and the causes of DIC.

10 To understand the principles of anticoagulant therapy with heparin and warfarin and to know about the laboratory control of such therapy.

11 To be aware of the natural anticoagulant mechanisms in blood and the concept of the pre-thrombotic state (thrombophilia).

Normal haemostasis

The cessation of bleeding following trauma to blood vessels results from three processes: (a) the contraction of vessel walls; (b) the formation of a platelet plug at the site of the break in the vessel wall; and (c) the formation of a fibrin clot. The clot forms within and around the platelet aggregates to form a firm haemostatic plug. The relative importance of these three processes probably varies according to the size of the vessels involved. Thus, in bleeding from a minor wound, the formation of a haemostatic plug is probably sufficient in itself, whereas, in larger vessels, contraction of the vessel walls also plays a part in haemostasis. The initial plug is formed almost entirely of platelets but this is friable and is subsequently stabilized by fibrin formation.

Classification of haemostatic defects

Although the action of platelets, the clotting mechanism and the integrity of the vascular wall are all closely related in the prevention of bleeding, it is convenient to consider that abnormalities in haemostasis arise from defects in one of these three processes. The commonest cause of bleeding is a deficiency of platelets; the second commonest cause is an abnormality in the clotting mechanism. The remaining patients bleed as a result of abnormal platelet function or vascular abnormalities.

A clinical distinction can frequently be made between bleeding due to clotting defects and bleeding due to a diminished number of platelets (Ingram 1977). Patients with clotting defects usually present with bleeding into deep tissues, that is, muscles or joints. On the other hand, patients with a deficiency of platelets usually present with superficial bleeding, that is, bleeding into the skin and from the epithelial surfaces of the nose, uterus and other organs. Haemorrhages into the skin include petechiae, which are less than 1 mm in diameter (Fig. 11.1) and ecchymoses, which are larger than petechiae and vary considerably in size (Fig. 11.2). A further useful clinical distinction is that bleeding usually persists from the time of injury in the case of platelet deficiency, since platelet numbers are inadequate to form a good platelet plug, whereas in clotting defects the initial bleeding may cease in the normal time since platelet plugs are readily formed, but as a consequence of the failure to form an adequate clot the platelet plug is not stabilized by fibrin formation and subsequently disintegrates, resulting in a delayed onset of prolonged bleeding. The clinical distinction is by no means complete, as deep-seated haemorrhage is sometimes found in platelet

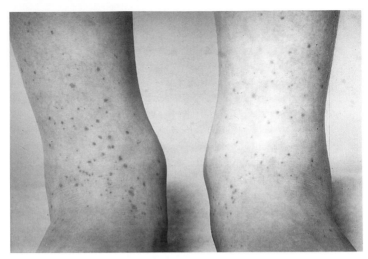

Fig. 11.1 Multiple pin-point haemorrhages (petechiae) on the legs of a patient with idiopathic autoimmune thrombocytopenic purpura.

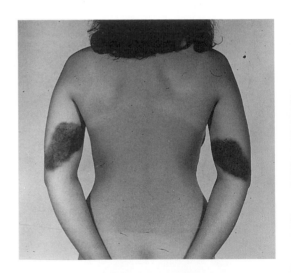

Fig. 11.2 Large ecchymoses on both upper arms of a woman with idiopathic autoimmune thrombocytopenic purpura.

deficiency and, on the other hand, superficial bleeding may occur in clotting defects.

Petechial haemorrhages and ecchymoses and bleeding from other sites may occur when the number of platelets falls below $80 \times 10^9/l$. At levels between 20 and $80 \times 10^9/l$, petechiae, ecchymoses and nose bleeds are the commonest symptoms, but below $20 \times 10^9/l$, gross haemorrhage (melaena, haematemesis, haematuria) becomes increasingly common. However, there is a great deal of variation in the relationship between the platelet count and haemorrhage in individual patients.

Platelets

MORPHOLOGY AND LIFE-SPAN

Platelets are discoid, non-nucleated, granule-containing cells (2–3 μm in diameter) that are formed in the bone marrow by the fragmentation of the cytoplasm of megakaryocytes. Their concentration in normal blood is $160–450 \times 10^9/l$.

The plasma membrane of a platelet contains glycoproteins (GP) that are important in the interaction of platelets with subendothelial connective tissue and other platelets. These include GP Ia which binds to collagen, GP Ib which binds to von Willebrand factor (VWF) and GP IIb/IIIa which binds to fibrinogen. The platelet membrane is extensively invaginated to form a surface-connected canalicular system through which the contents of platelet granules are released. Another intracellular membrane system known as the dense tubular system is rich in calcium, phospholipid-bound arachidonic acid, phospholipase A_2 (which mobilizes arachidonic acid), cyclo-oxygenase and thromboxane synthase and is the main site of prostaglandin and thromboxane synthesis. The platelet also contains contractile micro-filaments, an equatorial band of microtubules involved in maintaining its normal discoid shape and two main types of ultrastructurally identifiable granules. The α-granules, which are the most numerous, contain platelet factor 4 (heparin neutralizing factor), platelet-derived growth factor (which stimulates mitosis in vascular smooth muscle cells), VWF and fibrinogen. The contents of the dense granules (δ-granules) include adenosine triphosphate (ATP), adenosine disphosphate (ADP), 5-hydroxytryptamine (which causes vasoconstriction) and calcium.

The life-span of the platelet has been determined by labelling platelets *in vitro* with radioactive chromium (^{51}Cr) and studying their fate after reinjection into the circulation; it is of the order of 10 days.

PHYSIOLOGY

The main function of platelets is the formation of a haemostatic plug at sites of damage to vascular endothelium. First the platelets stick to exposed subendothelial collagen and microfibrils. Adhesion is potentiated by VWF, also known as Factor VIII-related antigen, present in plasma. VWF has two binding sites, one for glycoprotein Ib on the platelet and one for the microfibrils and can thus cross-link platelets to microfibrils. Within 1–2 seconds of adhesion, platelets change their shape from a disc to a more rounded form with spicules which encourage platelet–platelet interaction (aggregation) and they also release the contents of their granules (platelet release reaction). The most important substance released is ADP. The platelets are also stimulated to produce the prostaglandin, thromboxane A_2. The release of ADP and thromboxane A_2 causes an interaction of other platelets with the adherent platelets and with each other (secondary platelet aggregation), thus leading to the formation of a platelet plug. On the surface of activated platelets, glycoprotein IIb/IIIa undergoes a conformational change to provide binding sites for fibrinogen which plays a role in linking platelets together to form aggregates. It appears that prostacyclin released by endothelial and vascular smooth muscle cells inhibits platelet aggregation and may thus limit the extent of the platelet plug. Whereas thromboxane A_2 is a potent vasoconstrictor, prostacyclin is a powerful vasodilator.

At the site of injury, factor VII is activated by tissue factor of the intrinsic pathway (see Fig. 11.3) and initiates the formation of a fibrin clot within and around the platelet plug (p. 215). When platelets aggregate, certain phospholipids (platelet factor 3) are exposed on their surface which adsorb a number of clotting factors (VIII, IX, X, V) and thus considerably enhance the speed of the clotting reaction on and around the platelet surface. Platelets are also responsible for the contraction of the fibrin clot once it has been formed.

TESTS OF PLATELET FUNCTION

The bleeding time

The bleeding time is estimated by making small wounds in the skin of the forearm after applying a blood-pressure cuff to the upper arm and inflating to 40 mmHg; the average time that elapses until bleeding ceases is then measured. The wounds are three punctures made with a lancet in the method of Ivy, or one or two short incisions in the various template methods; the depth of the wound is standardized. The normal range depends on the method and is 2–4 minutes with the Ivy method. Since the wound only damages small vessels, haemostasis is mainly dependent on the formation of a platelet plug and hence the bleeding time is prolonged either when platelet numbers are reduced or when platelet function is impaired. It is almost always normal in the presence of clotting defects.

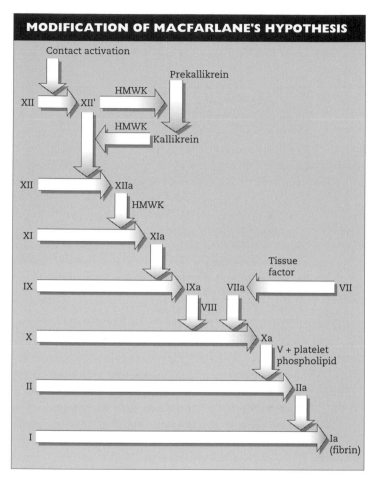

MODIFICATION OF MACFARLANE'S HYPOTHESIS

Fig. 11.3 Modification of MacFarlane's enzyme-cascade hypothesis regarding the sequence of reactions from surface contact to fibrin formation. The suffix 'a' denotes the enzymatically active form of each coagulation factor. HMWK, high molecular weight kininogen.

When platelet function is normal, there is a good correlation between the platelet count and the bleeding time (Harker & Slichter 1972). Bleeding times are not prolonged until the platelet count has fallen to $100 \times 10^9/l$. Below that value, there is a progressive and proportional prolongation in bleeding time, the time lengthening from the normal average of about 3 minutes to reach about 30 minutes as the platelet count falls to $10 \times 10^9/l$. Below $10 \times 10^9/l$, bleeding times may be prolonged to 1 hour or more.

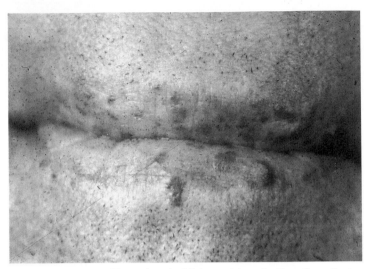

Fig. 11.4 Vascular malformations (reddish purple) on the lips of a patient with hereditary haemorrhagic telangiectasia; such lesions increase in number with advancing age. This rare condition is inherited as an autosomal dominant characteristic and may lead to recurrent gastrointestinal haemorrhage and chronic iron-deficiency anaemia.

On the other hand, when platelet function is impaired, bleeding times are longer than might be expected from platelet numbers (e.g. in uraemia, in von Willebrand's disease and after the ingestion of aspirin). The greatest value of the bleeding time is in detecting impaired platelet function in individuals with a normal platelet count.

Other tests

A large number of *in vitro* tests of platelet function have been described. The most commonly used tests study the aggregation of platelets following the addition of substances such as ADP, adrenaline, thrombin, collagen or ristocetin to platelet-rich plasma. Aggregation causes a decrease in optical density and the test is performed using special equipment capable of continuously recording optical density.

Thrombocytopenic and non-thrombocytopenic purpura

'Purpura' is the collective term for bleeding into the skin or mucous membranes. Patients with purpura can be separated into those with low platelet counts (thrombocytopenic) and those with normal platelet counts (non-thrombocytopenic). The non-thrombocytopenic group can be subdivided into those patients who have qualitative platelet defects and a larger group who have vascular abnormalities. The latter is a miscellaneous group and contains congenital disorders such as hereditary haemorrhagic telangiectasia (Fig. 11.4), the Ehlers–Danlos syndrome and acquired diseases such as Henoch–Schönlein purpura (allergic purpura), scurvy, purpura senilis and the purpura of infectious diseases. Purpura simplex (simple easy bruising), which may also be due to a vascular abnormality, is a common benign condition affecting otherwise healthy females of childbearing age.

Causes of thrombocytopenia

The mechanisms leading to thrombocytopenia are:
1 a failure of platelet production by the megakaryocytes;
2 a shortened life-span of the platelets, or
3 increased pooling of platelets in an enlarged spleen.
The distinction between the first two of these possibilities can be made by assessing the number of megakaryocytes in a marrow aspirate or trephine biopsy of the marrow.
The causes of thrombocytopenia are given in Table 11.1.

FAILURE OF PLATELET PRODUCTION

If megakaryocytes are few or absent, it may be assumed that platelet production is at fault. The bone-marrow smears may also reveal other features which indicate the nature of the disease if evidence has not already been obtained from the peripheral blood. Thus, there may be a generalized aplasia of the bone-marrow (aplastic anaemia) or a selective decrease in megakaryocytes caused by certain drugs (e.g. chlorothiazides, tolbutamide), alcoholism, and certain viruses (e.g. EB virus, measles, varicella, cytomegalovirus). (Shortened platelet survival mediated through immunological mechanisms is frequently more important than failure of platelet production in the pathogenesis of thrombocytopenia in viral infections.) Another cause of reduced platelet production is marked infiltration of the marrow by malignant cells (e.g. in leukaemia, lymphoma, myeloma and carcinoma) or by fibrous tissue. Reduced platelet production may also occur in patients with normal or increased numbers of megakaryocytes when there is ineffective megakaryocytopoiesis, as in severe vitamin B_{12} or folate deficiency or in myelodysplastic syndromes.

SHORTENED PLATELET SURVIVAL

If the megakaryocytes in the marrow are numerous, then the

THROMBOCYTOPENIA

FAILURE OF PLATELET PRODUCTION
Aplastic anaemia (p. 177)
Drugs, alcoholism
Viruses
Myelodysplasia
Paroxysmal nocturnal haemoglobinuria (p. 70)
Bone marrow infiltration (carcinoma, leukaemia, lymphoma, myeloma,
   myelofibrosis, storage diseases including Gaucher's disease,
   osteopetrosis)
Megaloblastic anaemia due to B_{12} or folate deficiency
Hereditary thrombocytopenia (e.g. thrombocytopenia with absent radii,
   gray-platelet syndrome, Bernard–Soulier syndrome, Wiskott–Aldrich
   syndrome)

SHORTENED PLATELET SURVIVAL
Immune
Idiopathic autoimmune thrombocytopenic purpura
Secondary autoimmune thrombocytopenic purpura (SLE and other
   collagen diseases, lymphoma, chronic lymphocytic leukaemia, HIV
   infection)
Drugs, alcoholism
Infections (viral, bacterial or parasitic)
Post-transfusion purpura
Neonatal alloimmune thrombocytopenia

Non-immune
Disseminated intravascular coagulation (p. 228), thrombotic
   thrombocytopenic purpura, haemolytic uraemic syndrome

INCREASED SPLENIC POOLING

Table 11.1 Some causes of thrombocytopenia.

thrombocytopenia is usually due to an excessive rate of removal of platelets from the peripheral circulation. In most cases the destruction results from autoantibodies attached to the platelet surface and the disease is termed 'autoimmune thrombocytopenic purpura'. Occasionally it is due to intravascular platelet consumption due to: (a) disseminated intravascular coagulation; or (b) interaction with damaged small blood vessels (microangiopathic thrombocytopenia) as in thrombotic thrombocytopenic purpura or the haemolytic uraemic syndrome.

Idiopathic autoimmune thrombocytopenic purpura (ITP)

ITP is characterized by petechiae (Fig. 11.1), bruising (Fig. 11.2), spontaneous bleeding from mucous membranes and a reduction in the plate-let count (without neutropenia or, usually, anaemia). The disease presents in both an acute and chronic form (Karpatkin 1980; Kirchner 1992). Patients with chronic ITP have autoantibodies in their plasma and on their platelets (Imbach 1994) which result in a shortened life-span due to premature destruction in the spleen. The antibodies are usually directed against the platelet glycoproteins IIb/IIIa or Ib. It is thought that acute ITP is caused by immune complexes rather than by platelet autoantibodies. However, there is evidence that autoantibodies against the platelet glycoproteins IIb/IIIa and Ib are also present in some patients with this condition. The platelet life-span is shortened in ITP, often reduced to about 1–2 days or less (e.g. 2 hours) compared to the normal life-span of 10 days. In approximately 30% of patients the destruction takes place only in the spleen, and in the rest it also occurs in the liver.

Clinical features
Acute ITP is seen at all ages but is most common before the age of 10 years. Two-thirds of patients give a history of a common childhood viral infection (e.g. upper respiratory tract infection, chicken pox, measles) 2–3 weeks preceding the purpura. Platelet counts are often less than 20 × 10^9/l. In most patients the disease runs a self-limiting course of 2–4 weeks but in approximately 20% it becomes chronic, that is, lasts more than 6 months. The disease is almost always self-limiting when there is a history of preceding infection. The mortality is low, the main danger being intracranial bleeding.

Chronic ITP occurs mainly in the age period 15–50 years; it has a higher incidence in women than in men. The chronic form is usually not severe and mortality is low; platelet counts are usually between 20 and 80 × 10^9/l. Spontaneous cures are rare and the disease is characterized by relapses and remissions. In a large series, about one-third of the patients with chronic ITP had petechiae and ecchymoses as the only presenting signs (Doan et al. 1960). The remainder also had bleeding from the following sites in decreasing order of frequency: nose, gums, vagina (menorrhagia), gastrointestinal and renal tract. Cerebral haemorrhage occurred in 3%. As a general rule the spleen is not palpable.

Diagnosis
In idiopathic thrombocytopenia, bone marrow megakaryocytes are increased in number (up to four- or eight-fold) and in size. An absence or reduction of megakaryocytes rules out the idiopathic disease. The

marrow aspiration also serves to exclude other causes of thrombocytopenia, such as aplastic anaemia, leukaemia or marrow infiltration by carcinoma cells, lymphoma cells or myeloma cells. Thrombocytopenia is sometimes the first sign of systemic lupus erythematosus (SLE). Thrombocytopenia due to drugs must also be excluded.

Treatment

In acute ITP, over 80% recover without any treatment. Corticosteroids are widely used; they increase the platelet count and so reduce the duration of thrombocytopenia. High-doses of intravenous Ig cause a rapid increase in the platelet count and are administered, with or without corticosteroids, to children with severe thrombocytopenia or life-threatening haemorrhage.

High-dose corticosteroid therapy increases the platelet count to more than $50 \times 10^9/l$ and, usually, more than $100 \times 10^9/l$ in two-thirds of patients with chronic ITP. Adults are often started on prednisolone 60 mg/day and the dosage reduced gradually after a remission is achieved, or after 4 weeks. However, in only a third of patients who initially have a complete remission, is the remission long-lived.

Splenectomy should be considered if the response to corticosteroids is poor, the minimum dose of corticosteroid required to prevent bleeding is unacceptably high or a patient relapses after responding to corticosteroids. About 75% of the patients respond fully to splenectomy, usually within 1 week. However, 10–15% of complete responders will relapse after an interval.

Azathioprine or cyclophosphamide can be used in patients who fail to respond to splenectomy, in an attempt to reduce antibody formation. These drugs have been reported to be effective in some cases.

High doses of intravenous Ig (e.g. 400 mg/kg/day for 5 days) have also been found to increase the platelet count to greater than $50 \times 10^9/l$ in 80% of patients with chronic ITP and to normal values in greater than 50%. However, the increase is usually transient; the platelet count returns to pre-treatment levels in 2–6 weeks. Ig probably acts by interfering with platelet destruction by inhibiting the binding of the Fc portion of the IgG antibodies on the platelet surface to Fc receptors on macrophages.

Secondary autoimmune thrombocytopenic purpura

An autoimmune thrombocytopenia may precede other manifestations of SLE by several years and may complicate the course of SLE, other autoimmune disorders, lymphoma and chronic lymphocytic leukaemia. Patients infected with the human immunodeficiency virus (HIV) may

develop either autoimmune thrombocytopenia or immune thrombocytopenia (caused by immune complexes) long before developing
other characteristic features.

Drug-induced immune thrombocytopenia

Certain drugs such as heparin, gold salts, quinine, quinidine, sulphonamides or penicillin cause a shortening of platelet life-span in a small
proportion of recipients by an immunological mechanism. The drug (e.g.
quinine or quinidine) binds to the platelet membrane, and antibody
formed against the drug–platelet complex combines with platelets that
have reacted with the drug but not with normal platelets. Heparin causes
thrombocytopenia in 1–3% of recipients by a variation of this mechanism:
the drug binds to α-granule-derived platelet factor 4 on the platelet
surface and the resulting immune complexes combine with the Fc
receptors of platelets causing platelet activation and, in some cases,
thrombosis.

Other immune thrombocytopenias

In the rare condition known as *post-transfusion purpura* severe
thrombocytopenia develops 5–8 days after a transfusion, as a result of the
destruction of the recipient's platelets. Platelet-specific alloantibodies are
present in the serum but the explanation for the destruction of the patient's own platelets is unclear.

Transient but potentially serious *neonatal alloimmune thrombocytopenia*
may occur in babies of healthy mothers. The mother forms IgG
alloantibodies against a fetal platelet-specific antigen lacking in the mother's platelets and inherited from the father; these antibodies cross the
placenta and damage fetal platelets (analogous to haemolytic disease of
the newborn, p. 252).

**Thrombotic thrombocytopenic purpura and
haemolytic uraemic syndrome**

Thrombotic thrombocytopenic purpura is a serious illness of unknown
aetiology characterized by fever and widespread arteriolar platelet
thrombi leading to fragmentation of red cells, thrombocytopenia, neurological symptoms and renal impairment. The haemolytic uraemic syndrome is a similar disorder affecting infants, young children and the
elderly in which the arteriolar thrombi are more-or-less limited to the
kidneys. In some patients, the disease follows a bout of diarrhoea caused
by verotoxin-producing *Escherichia coli*.

INCREASED SPLENIC POOLING

A normal spleen contains within its microcirculation about 30% of all the blood platelets; the platelets in the splenic pool exchange freely with those in the general circulation. The splenic platelet pool increases with increasing splenic size so that in patients with moderate to massive splenomegaly it may account for 50–90% of all blood platelets, thus causing thrombocytopenia. Another factor contributing to the thrombocytopenia in patients with splenomegaly is an increase in plasma volume (p. 73).

Abnormalities of platelet function

These must be suspected in any patient with non-thrombocytopenic purpura. An acquired defect of platelet function is found after aspirin ingestion and after therapy with sulphinpyrazone (a competitive inhibitor of cyclo-oxygenase) or dipyridamole (Persantin). Aspirin has a moderate effect on the bleeding time: 2 hours after the ingestion of 600 mg of aspirin, the bleeding time rises above the normal range in 30% of subjects and may be as long as 20 minutes. This prolongation is sufficient to provoke abnormal bleeding in certain people and aspirin is contraindicated in those with bleeding disorders. Aspirin acts by irreversibly acetylating cyclo-oxygenase and this inhibits thromboxane A_2 synthesis with a subsequent reduction in platelet aggregation. The effect of a single dose of aspirin can be detected for 1 week, i.e. until most of the platelets present at the time of taking the aspirin have been replaced by newly formed platelets.

Various abnormalities of platelet function may also be found after treatment with other drugs such as some non-steroidal anti-inflammatory drugs (e.g. indomethacin or ibuprofen), penicillin, cephalosporins, dextrans and heparin (high doses) and after the consumption of alcohol.

Other causes of an acquired abnormality of platelet function include chronic myeloproliferative disorders (p. 164), myelodysplastic syndromes, paraproteinaemias (e.g. myeloma or Waldenström's macroglobulinaemia) and uraemia.

Inherited disorders of platelet function are very rare and include:

1 Bernard–Soulier syndrome (autosomal recessive inheritance) in which there is a deficiency of glycoprotein Ib in the platelet membrane and there are giant platelets;

2 Glanzmann's thrombasthenia (autosomal recessive inheritance) in

Continued

which there is a deficiency of glycoprotein IIb/IIIa in the platelet membrane and platelets are normal in morphology and number;
3 δ-storage pool disease (dense granule deficiency) and grey platelet syndrome (α-granule deficiency), and
4 defects of thromboxane synthesis, including cyclo-oxygenase deficiency and thromboxane synthase deficiency.

Platelet transfusions

It is often possible to raise the platelet count temporarily by platelet transfusions. The main indication for platelet transfusion is severe haemorrhage caused by: (a) thrombocytopenia due to diminished platelet production or disseminated intravascular coagulation; or (b) abnormal platelet function. Transfusion may also be indicated in a patient with thrombocytopenia or defective platelet function prior to surgery (p. 252). Another indication for platelet transfusion is thrombocytopenia (platelets $< 50 \times 10^9/l$) in patients receiving massive blood transfusions (p. 243); blood stored for 48 hours has virtually no viable platelets. When thrombocytopenia results from excess destruction caused by platelet antibodies, the response to transfusion is poor. Platelets are transfused as platelet concentrates and should be given within 5 days of withdrawal from the donor (p. 252). In order to prevent *spontaneous* haemorrhage, platelet counts need only be maintained above $20 \times 10^9/l$ since severe bleeding is rare above this level.

Normal coagulation mechanism

The mechanisms involved in the clotting cascade were elucidated in the period 1950–1970, largely by the work of MacFarlane and his colleagues (1964, 1969). The essential feature of the cascade is the presence of a number of steps activated in sequence. Each step is characterized by the conversion of a proenzyme into an enzyme by the splitting of one or more peptide bonds, which brings about a conformational change in the molecule and reveals the active enzyme site.

There are two pathways or systems present within the cascade. First, there is the intrinsic system, all the components of which are in the plasma. The sequence of action of factors in the intrinsic system is XII, XI, IX (with VIII as cofactor), X, II and I, as illustrated in Fig. 11.3. The clotting sequence is initiated by the adsorption of factor XII to negatively charged subendothelial collagen and microfibrils which results in the appearance of an active enzyme site on the molecule. Following limited activation, factor XII converts the plasma protein prekallikrein to kallikrein which in turn activates factor XII fully to XIIa. Another plasma protein, high molecular weight kininogen, is a non-enzymatic accelerator of these interactions. Factor XIIa then acts on XI to form the active enzyme XIa. The intrinsic system can also become activated by different mechanisms, namely by the activation of factor IX by factor VIIa of the extrinsic system and by the activation of factor XI by thrombin. These are clearly important mechanisms, as people with a deficiency of factor XII do not have a significant bleeding tendency. Factor XIa then acts on IX to form IXa which then acts on X to form Xa, using factor VIII as a cofactor. Factor Xa then acts on factor II (prothrombin), using factor V as a cofactor to form factor IIa (thrombin). Factor IIa splits several small negatively charged peptide fragments from factor I (fibrinogen), thus removing repulsive forces from the molecule and allowing the remainder to polymerize and form the fibrin fibre. Finally, factor XIIIa, generated by the activation of factor XIII by thrombin, stabilizes and strengthens the fibrin polymers by forming covalent bonds between the fibrin chains (glutamine–lysine bridges).

The interaction of factors IX, VIII and X, takes place mainly on the surface of platelets, where the rate of reaction is very considerably increased when compared to the rate occurring in solution. Hence bleeding in thrombocytopenia results from a failure of the clotting cascade as well as the lack of a platelet plug.

Secondly, there is the extrinsic system which consists of two factors: tissue factor (also known as factor III or tissue thromboplastin) which is released from damaged tissue; and factor VII, present in the serum as an inactive serine esterase. Following trauma, tissue factor and factor VII form a complex, factor VII becomes activated and then acts on X to form Xa. Both systems thus share a final common path (factor X, II and I).

Calcium is required at several stages in the two systems.

Six of the synonyms for the factors are still in general use and should be known. They are: anti-haemophilic globulin, VIII; Christmas factor, IX; prothrombin, II; thrombin, IIa; fibrinogen, I; and fibrin, Ia.

Apart from the basic reactions mentioned above, there are additional interactions between various components of the coagulation mechanism, mainly in the form of positive and negative feedback systems. Thus, factors activated late in the sequence potentiate reactions at earlier stages (for instance, factor IIa potentiates the activity of factors VIII and V).

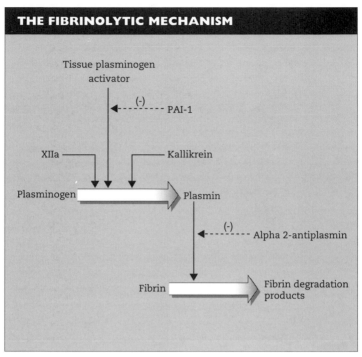

THE FIBRINOLYTIC MECHANISM

Tissue plasminogen activator

(-) ------ PAI-1

XIIa ——— Kallikrein

Plasminogen ⟹ Plasmin

(-) ------ Alpha 2-antiplasmin

Fibrin ⟹ Fibrin degradation products

Fig. 11.5 The fibrinolytic mechanism. The white arrows indicate conversion, the continuous lines activity, the broken lines inhibition. PAI-1, plasminogen activator inhibitor-1.

The fibrinolytic mechanism

The complex mechanism for producing fibrin is counterbalanced by a mechanism for the enzymatic lysis of clots (Fig. 11.5). The dissolution of the fibrin into fibrin-degradation products (FDP) is carried out by the proteolytic plasma enzyme plasmin. Plasmin is present in the plasma in an inactive form, plasminogen, which is synthesized in the liver; plasminogen is converted to plasmin mainly by tissue plasminogen activator (t-PA), which is synthesized and released by the vascular endothelium. There may also be a limited activation of plasminogen by factor XIIa and kallikrein. Bradykinin, which is released from high molecular weight kininogen by the action of kallikrein, is a powerful stimulator of t-PA release. The plasma contains a physiological inhibitor of t-PA known as plasminogen activator inhibitor-1 (PAI-1). Activated protein C (p. 233) inactivates PAI-1 and thereby stimulates fibrinolysis.

Plasmin is not specific for fibrin but can also break down other protein components of plasma, including fibrinogen and the clotting factors V and VIII, and thus the following mechanism is present which confines the activities of plasmin to fibrin.

When fibrin is formed, t-PA and plasminogen are specifically adsorbed onto fibrin; the t-PA–fibrin complex has a high infinity for plasminogen and converts it to plasmin, which digests the fibrin to which it is adsorbed. Under normal conditions, any plasmin released from the fibrin into the circulation is immediately inactivated by combining with the liver-derived plasma inhibitor, α_2-antiplasmin. In this way, generalized breakdown of fibrinogen and other proteins does not occur.

As well as tissue activator, physiological activators of plasminogen are present in many body secretions, especially in urine (urokinase) and in the pleural and peritoneal cavities. Urokinase and recombinant plasminogen activator injected intravenously or into the coronary artery are useful therapeutic agents for the treatment of early acute myocardial infarction. These drugs may also be useful in other types of thrombosis. Non-physiological activators, such as streptokinase, derived from certain streptococci, and acylated plasminogen–streptokinase activator complex (Apsac) are also being used as thrombolytic agents.

Tests for clotting defects

There are three basic tests which are widely used:

1   the *activated partial thromboplastin time* (e.g. kaolin–cephalin clotting time) which estimates the activity of the intrinsic system;

2   the *prothrombin time* which estimates the activity of the extrinsic system, and

3   the *thrombin time* (p. 229) which is prolonged when there is an inherited or acquired deficiency of fibrinogen, or an inherited or acquired abnormal fibrinogen molecule (dysfibrinogenaemia) or in the presence of heparin or raised levels of fibrin degradation products.

Patients with clotting defects fall into two groups; in the first, and by far the largest group, are those patients with liver disease or DIC who have acquired deficiencies of several factors in both the extrinsic and intrinsic pathways, and patients with acquired deficiencies of factors II, VII, IX and X (vitamin K-dependent factors) resulting from treatment with coumarin drugs or from vitamin K deficiency (p. 227). It can be seen from Fig. 11.5 that three of the vitamin K-dependent factors (II, VII and X) lie in the extrinsic system. Therefore, this first group of patients will have a prolonged prothrombin time. In the second and much smaller group are patients with congenital defects of one of the clotting factors.

There are several recognized congenital clotting defects, but 80–90% of the patients in this group are haemophiliacs (factor VIII deficiency). About 10–20% have factor IX deficiency, and only about 1% have deficiencies of one of the other eight factors. Thus in practice, almost all the congenital deficiencies involve factors in the initial stages of the intrinsic system, and these can be detected by abnormalities in the activated partial thromboplastin time (APTT). By carrying out both the APTT and the prothrombin time tests, it is therefore possible to determine whether the defect lies in the initial stages of the intrinsic system or in the components comprising the extrinsic system. If both tests are abnormal, then the defect is in the final common path or there are multiple abnormalities.

TEST FOR THE INTRINSIC SYSTEM

Activated partial thromboplastin time (APTT)

There is a wide range in the time taken for venous blood to clot in a glass tube at 37°C. This wide range in the whole-blood clotting time is due to two variables. First, activation of factor XII by the glass surface is variable and depends on such factors as the type of glass. Secondly, there is a variation in the coagulation potentiating activities supplied by the platelets, as platelet numbers vary considerably between individuals. The variation due to these two factors can be substantially abolished by the addition of kaolin and a phospholipid (partial thromboplastin). Kaolin provides a maximal stimulus for factor XII activation and the phospholipid acts as a platelet substitute. The test is simple to carry out. Citrated plasma is obtained and to this is added a mixture of kaolin and phospholipid followed by calcium, and the time taken for the mixture to clot is measured. Prolongation of the clotting time is almost always due to deficiency of factors VIII and IX (provided that deficiency of factor X onwards has been excluded by the prothrombin time) and the test is sufficiently sensitive to detect deficiencies of both these factors when their concentration is reduced to 30% or less of the normal value; that is, it will detect the mild haemophiliacs who only have severe bleeding after minor surgical procedures.

If the APTT is prolonged, it is possible to confirm the diagnosis of either factor VIII or IX deficiency if plasma is available from known cases of haemophilia and factor IX deficiency. Thus, if the addition of plasma known to be deficient only in factor VIII does not shorten the clotting time of the sample from the patient under investigation, then the patient must also have a deficiency of factor VIII. Specialized tests are also available for measuring fairly precisely the levels of factor VIII and IX, expressed as a percentage of the normal value; these tests should always be carried out in appropriate cases.

TEST FOR THE EXTRINSIC SYSTEM

The prothrombin time

The test used to measure the integrity of the extrinsic system is the one-stage prothrombin time (PT). This test is carried out by adding tissue thromboplastin derived from brain (tissue factor, factor III) together with calcium to citrated plasma. Reference to Fig. 11.3 shows that tissue factor feeds into the intrinsic system at the stage X → Xa and hence prolongation of the prothrombin time results from deficiencies of I, II, V, VII and X. The prothrombin time is thus a misnomer since deficiency of at least five factors affects the test and prothrombin deficiency alone must be gross before the prothrombin time is prolonged. The test is chiefly sensitive to deficiency of factors V, VII and X. A deficiency of platelets does not affect the prothrombin time.

When measuring the prothrombin time and APTT, it is necessary simultaneously to determine the clotting time using a lyophilized control plasma. This is because there are always small differences in the activities of the reagents that are used.

When the prothrombin time is used for the control of oral anticoagulant therapy, the results are expressed as the international normalized ratio (INR). This is derived from the prothrombin time ratio (i.e. patient's prothrombin time/mean normal prothrombin time) and a factor determined for each thromboplastin reagent by comparing its activity against an international reference preparation. The value of using the INR is that the same therapeutic ranges apply irrespective of the source of thromboplastin.

Congenital coagulation disorders

Blood clotting abnormalities can be conveniently divided into two categories, the congenital defects and the acquired defects. This section deals with those that are present from birth.

There is a group of patients who complain of excessive bleeding, either spontaneous or following trauma, usually starting early in life, and who frequently have a family history of a similar condition. These patients usually have one of three diseases, namely, haemophilia, factor IX deficiency or von Willebrand's disease.

HAEMOPHILIA (FACTOR VIII DEFICIENCY, HAEMOPHILIA A)

The term 'haemophilia', first used by Schönlein in 1839, was applied to a life-long tendency to prolonged haemorrhage found in males and dependent on the transmission of a sex-linked abnormal gene. During the decade 1950–60, it was found that there are in fact two diseases within the group of patients who, on clinical and genetic grounds, had been diagnosed as having haemophilia: patients with factor VIII deficiency, and those with factor IX deficiency. The term haemophilia has been retained for factor VIII deficiency, as this is the more common deficiency; the terms 'factor IX deficiency', 'haemophilia B' or 'Christmas disease' (after the name of the first patient) are used for the other disease.

Genetics, prevalence and biochemistry

Deficiency of factor VIII results from an abnormality in the factor VIII gene which lies at the tip of the long arm of the X chromosome (Kazazian 1993). Various abnormalities in the nucleotide sequence of this gene have been identified in a number of cases of haemophilia, ranging from single point mutations to large deletions. The disease is almost entirely confined to males (XY) since the normal X chromosome in heterozygous females is almost always capable of bringing about adequate factor VIII production. The prevalence of this disorder is about 1 per 10000 males. Females with haemophilia have been observed extremely rarely and these are either homozygotes for the abnormal gene or are heterozygotes in whom the normal X chromosome has not produced sufficient quantities of factor VIII due to Lyonization. Daughters of males with haemophilia are obligatory carriers of the gene, since they must inherit the abnormal X chromosome. Sons, on the other hand, are always normal, since they inherit the Y chromosome. A female with a genetic defect on one X chromosome will transmit the disease to half her sons, and half her daughters will become carriers. Patients suspected of having haemophilia should be carefully questioned for a history of a bleeding disorder occurring in the relations on the maternal side as opposed to the paternal side. There is a steady spontaneous mutation rate of the gene responsible for factor VIII production, since approximately one-third of all haemophiliacs have no family history of the disease and this has been corroborated from studies on the genomic DNA.

The factor VIII molecule is a protein with a molecular weight of 8×10^4 daltons. In the plasma, factor VIII is only found complexed with VWF, which acts as a carrier and prolongs its plasma half-life. Moreover, factor VIII has coagulant activity only when combined with VWF. The factor VIII coagulant activity can be measured biologically by its ability to act as a

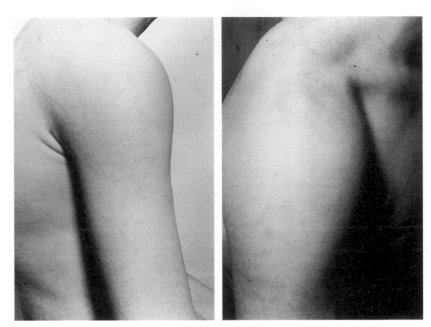

Fig. 11.6 Haemarthrosis of the shoulder joint in a patient with haemophilia A.

cofactor to factor IXa (see Fig. 11.3); the VWF can be measured by
reaction with specific antibodies and is, therefore, also known as
factor VIII-related antigen. Although factor VIII coagulant activity is
greatly depressed in haemophilia, the amount of VWF is within normal
limits.

Detection of carriers and antenatal diagnosis (Kazazian 1993)

Female carriers on average have half the clotting activity per unit of VWF
compared to normal. Discrimination, however, is not perfect and in
about 10% of carriers the ratio between the clotting activity and VWF
content falls within the normal range; thus, those with abnormal ratios
can definitely be said to be carriers, but putative carriers with normal
ratios cannot be definitely assured that they do not have the abnormal
gene. Restriction fragment length polymorphisms (RFLP) linked to the
factor VIII gene and various genetic probes allow carriers to be identified
with better accuracy.

Prenatal diagnosis of haemophilia can be made by analysis of fetal
DNA or blood. DNA can be obtained either by chorionic villus sampling
between 9 and 12 weeks of gestation or by amniocentesis between 13
and 16 weeks. The presence or absence of the abnormal gene can be

BLEEDING SITES	
Lesion or operation	Percentage
Haemarthroses	79
Muscle haematomas	15
Haematuria	
Epistaxes	
Gastrointestinal bleeding	Each about 1–2%
Dental extraction	Total 6%
Major surgery	

Table 11.2 Frequency of bleeding sites in 207 haemophiliacs. (From Rizza 1977.)

established either directly using DNA probes for specific defects or indirectly by RFLP analysis. Fetal blood sampling is done between 18 and 20 weeks. Factor VIII levels are determined in the fetal plasma either on the basis of immunological reactivity or coagulation activity.

Clinical features

The characteristic clinical feature of severe haemophilia (Hoyer 1994) is the occurrence of spontaneous bleeding into joints (Fig. 11.6) and less frequently into muscles; these two sites account for about 95% of all bleeds requiring treatment (Table 11.2). The presenting symptom is pain in the affected area and this can be very severe. Haemophiliacs rapidly become expert at diagnosing the onset of haemorrhage in its earliest stages, allowing treatment to be initiated at a time when it can be most effective. If not properly treated, bleeding into joints results in crippling deformity. The knees, elbows and ankles are most commonly affected. Haematuria, epistaxis and gastrointestinal bleeding are less common. Intracranial bleeding is the most common cause of death from the disease itself, accounting for 25–30% of all such deaths; only about one-half of the affected patients have a history of trauma (Eyster et al. 1978).

The severity of bleeding and mode of presentation is related to the level of plasma factor VIII (Rizza 1977); this relationship is shown in Table 11.3. The severity of the disease often remains constant throughout a family.

Because of treatment with HIV-contaminated factor VIII concentrates between about 1978 and 1985, over 50% of patients with severe haemophilia in the United States and Europe became HIV-positive; many of these have died of the acquired immune deficiency syndrome (AIDS). In addition, virtually all haemophiliacs have been infected with hepatitis C virus (p. 247) due to treatment with non-virally inactivated factor concentrates.

FACTOR VIII LEVEL AND BLEEDING

Factor VIII level (units/100 ml)	Bleeding symptoms
50	None
25–50	Excessive bleeding after major surgery or serious accident (often not diagnosed until incident occurs)
5–25	Excessive bleeding after minor surgery and injuries
1–5	Severe bleeding after minor surgery (sometimes spontaneous haemorrhage)
0	Spontaneous bleeding into muscles and joints

Table 11.3 Relation between plasma factor VIII levels and severity of bleeding. (From Rizza 1977.)

Diagnosis

The diagnosis of haemophilia is strongly suggested by the laboratory finding of a normal extrinsic clotting system (normal prothrombin time) and a prolonged activated partial thromboplastin time. Confirmation can be obtained by showing that the addition of plasma from a known case of factor VIII deficiency to the patient's plasma does not correct the clotting defect or, can be obtained by a specific assay of factor VIII coagulant activity.

Treatment

Treatment should be given at the earliest sign of spontaneous or post-traumatic bleeding. It should also be given prophylactically if any type of operation is contemplated. Treatment consists of intravenous injections of freeze-dried factor VIII concentrate to maintain plasma factor VIII coagulant activity to between 5 and 100% of normal, depending on the severity of the injury or extent of the proposed surgical procedure. In general, the more extensive the bleeding or the degree of trauma, the larger the dose of factor VIII concentrate that is required. HIV has been virtually eliminated from currently used freeze-dried factor VIII preparations by using donors who do not have HIV antibodies and by heat-treating the final product at 80°C for 72 hours, a process known to kill the virus.

Freeze-dried factor VIII concentrates can be stored at 4°C and can be injected in adequate amounts in a small volume. This has made it possible for many patients to be treated at home, sometimes by self-administration, thus allowing factor VIII to be injected as soon as symptoms appear. Such early therapy results in both rapid cessation of bleeding and rapid recovery (Rizza & Spooner 1977).

Since the half-life of factor VIII in the plasma is about 12 hours, this factor has to be injected twice a day. Frequent assays of factor VIII levels in the plasma may be necessary to ensure that the concentration is being maintained at the appropriate level.

Approximately 5–10% of haemophiliac patients who are repeatedly injected with factor VIII develop antibodies which inhibit its functional activity. These patients require large amounts of factor VIII, or recourse may have to be made to the use of factor VIII of bovine or porcine origin. However the latter can only be used for a short time, since antibodies to these molecules develop rapidly.

The administration of factor VIII may be avoided in mild to moderate haemophilia by using the vasopressin analogue desmopressin (DDAVP) which causes a temporary increase in factor VIII clotting activity by provoking the release of factor VIII from endothelial cells. DDAVP is used intravenously or as snuff. The antifibrinolytic drug tranexamic acid should be administered with DDAVP as the latter also causes release of t-PA from the endothelium.

FACTOR IX DEFICIENCY (HAEMOPHILIA B, CHRISTMAS DISEASE)

The differentiation of factor IX deficiency from haemophilia due to lack of factor VIII was first made by Biggs and colleagues (1952). The clinical features and inheritance of factor IX deficiency are identical to those in factor VIII deficiency, but in general the disease is milder. Factor IX deficiency affects about 1 in every 50 000 males (i.e. is less frequent than factor VIII deficiency).

The APTT is prolonged and the PT normal. The diagnosis can be made by assay of the factor IX level. A freeze-dried factor IX concentrate (actually a prothrombin-complex concentrate containing factors II, VII, IX and X) is available and should be administered intravenously as soon as spontaneous or post-traumatic bleeding starts. Alternatively, fresh-frozen plasma may be used. Factor IX has a longer half-life in the plasma (24 hours) than factor VIII and hence can be given at less frequent intervals. It has been found that home treatment with factor IX as soon as bleeding starts, considerably reduces the need for hospital care.

VON WILLEBRAND'S DISEASE

The prevalence of this disease is greater than that of factor VIII de-ficiency. It was described by von Willebrand in 1926 as occurring in several families on islands in the Baltic (Åland Islands). It differs from haemophilia in that the defect is not sex-linked but usually inherited as an autosomal dominant character with varying expression. It is characterized by mild to severe bleeding. The bleeding results from either an abnormality or a deficiency of VWF (Lethagen 1993; Rick 1994). This factor is a protein with a molecular weight of 2.7×10^5 daltons and exists in the plasma as a variable-sized polymer ranging from a dimer to a molecule containing 50–100 subunits. It has a dual function: first, it is an adhesive molecule which binds platelets to subendothelial tissues; secondly, it acts as a carrier for factor VIII, one factor VIII molecule being associated with about 1000 VWF subunits. The reduction in VWF results in a reduction in factor VIII concentration (usually measured as clotting activity), which may be as low as 5–30% of normal, similar to that found in mild haemophilia. The excessive bleeding in the disease is thus due both to the failure of the platelets to adhere as well as to factor VIII deficiency. An additional finding is that, whereas the antibiotic ristocetin induces platelet aggregation in platelet-rich plasma from normal subjects, it fails to do so in platelet-rich plasma from people with severe von Willebrand's disease. This observation is the basis of a useful laboratory test for the diagnosis of this disease.

The gene for VWF is present on chromosome 12 and analysis of both the gene and the VWF protein have shown that there is considerable heterogeneity in the structural abnormalities found in von Willebrand's disease. Most abnormalities result in a simple quantitative reduction in VWF plasma concentration but many different qualitative defects in the molecule also occur.

Most patients are heterozygous for the von Willebrand gene and the extent of bleeding is not great. Spontaneous bleeding is usually confined to mucous membranes and skin and takes the form of epistaxes and ecchymoses. Severe haemorrhage may occur following surgical procedures. Bleeding into joints and muscles is rare except in patients who are homozygous for the defective gene.

The laboratory findings include a prolonged bleeding time, a prolonged APTT, reduced factor VIII clotting activity, reduced levels of VWF (factor VIII-related antigen or VW antigen) and impaired ristocetin-induced platelet aggregation; however, there may be periods when the bleeding time is within normal limits. The prolonged bleeding time distinguishes von Willebrand's disease from haemophilia and factor IX deficiency.

For mildly or moderately affected patients, desmopressin (DDAVP), which increases plasma levels of both VWF and factor VIII, should be considered before using blood products (Rodeghiero et al. 1991). Intermediate-purity factor VIII concentrates which contain VWF and factor

VIII are effective in stopping haemorrhage, mainly by correcting the bleeding time but also by increasing factor VIII clotting activity, which continues to increase for many hours after treatment. High-purity factor VIII concentrates are less effective than intermediate-purity concentrates since they have less effect on the bleeding time.

DEFICIENCY OF OTHER CLOTTING FACTORS

Single deficiencies of factors other than VIII and IX are very rare, but all possible deficiencies have been found and all except factor XII deficiency give rise to bleeding disorders of varying degrees of severity. The explanation for the absence of excessive haemorrhage in factor XII deficiency is that the activation of the intrinsic pathway can be initiated in the absence of factor XII by the activation of factor IX by factor VIIa of the extrinsic system and of factor XI by thrombin.

Acquired coagulation disorders

The hepatocytes are the major cell type involved in the synthesis of all the coagulation factors except factor VIII. Hence, severe liver disease may result in bleeding due both to a deficiency of several coagulation factors and to an abnormality in the structure and function of fibrinogen. In addition, liver disease may result in impaired clearance of activated clotting factors or t-PA leading to disseminated intravascular coagulation or increased fibrinolysis, respectively.

The final stages in the synthesis of factors II, VII, IX and X (collectively known as the prothrombin group or complex) involves a vitamin K-dependent carboxylase, which adds carboxyl (-COOH) groups to the proteins; these groups are necessary for the efficient functioning of the molecules.

The coumarin drugs are vitamin K antagonists and their administration results in only partial carboxylation of the prothrombin group of coagulation factors, which are consequently considerably less active than normal in the clotting cascade. Similar abnormalities are seen in vitamin K deficiency, which may be found in the newborn (haemorrhagic disease of the newborn), in patients with intestinal malabsorption and, since bile salts are required for vitamin K absorption, also in patients with biliary obstruction or biliary fistulae. Examination of Fig. 11.3 shows that, except for factor IX, the clotting factors involved are in the extrinsic system and hence the test that is used for detecting these acquired deficiencies is the prothrombin time.

DISSEMINATED INTRAVASCULAR COAGULATION

DIC describes a process in which there is a generalized activation of the clotting system followed by marked activation of the fibrinolytic system (Baker 1989; Muller-Berghaus 1989; Bick 1994). Acute DIC may be associated with premature separation of the placenta (abruptio placentae), amniotic fluid embolism or shock and may also be seen in certain bacterial infections such as meningococcaemia, where the endotoxin causes damage to monocytes and vascular endothelium. It is a common complication following intravascular haemolysis of red cells after a mismatched transfusion. The syndrome also occurs occasionally after extensive accidental or surgical trauma, particularly following thoracic operations. Chronic DIC is seen when there is retention of a dead fetus as well as in patients with disseminated carcinoma, lymphoma, leukaemia (especially acute promyelocytic leukaemia). Other clinical associations of DIC include purpura fulminans (following scarlet fever, chicken pox or rubella), brain injuries, extensive burns, liver disease and snake bites.

In those diseases that are associated with DIC, the clotting cascade may be activated in one or both of two ways, namely, by the binding and activation of factors XII and XI by damaged vascular endothelium and, by the release of tissue factor (tissue thromboplastin) from damaged tissues, monocytes or red cells. Dissemination of factors XIIa, XIa and III in the plasma leads to generalized fibrin deposition on vascular endothelium. If this is sufficiently extensive, there is a reduction of plasma fibrinogen concentration and other clotting factors, which impairs haemostatic activity. As a consequence of the fibrin formation, the fibrinolytic mechanism is activated (p. 217) resulting in high concentrations of FDP. This leads to further haemostatic impairment, since FDP inhibit fibrin clot formation by interfering with the polymerization of fibrin monomer. The FDP also interfere with the aggregation of platelets. The end result is generalized haemorrhage due to failure of the haemostatic mechanisms. The haemorrhagic manifestations may be mild or moderate in chronic DIC but may be so severe in acute DIC as to lead to death. They include petechiae, ecchymoses and bleeding from the nose, mouth, urinary and gastrointestinal tracts and vagina. Haemorrhage may also occur into the pituitary gland, liver, adrenals and brain.

As explained above, the usual clinical manifestation of the generalized activation of the clotting and fibrinolytic systems is haemorrhage. However, occasionally, activation of the clotting mechanism dominates over activation of fibrinolysis and the clinical picture is then that of widespread thrombosis and infarction; thrombi are most frequently found in the microvasculature. Mild hypotension is commonly present in acute DIC and may progress to become more severe and irreversible if not treated in time. Some patients with chronic DIC are asymptomatic because the activation of the clotting and fibrinolytic systems is finely balanced and the production of clotting factors and platelets is sufficiently increased to compensate for their increased consumption.

Diagnosis

This is partly dependent on being aware of the conditions with which DIC is associated. The investigations of value in the diagnosis of acute or chronic DIC are as follows.

1 *The platelet count.* Platelets become enmeshed in the fibrin clots on the vascular endothelium and thrombocytopenia is an early and very common sign.

2 *The activated partial thromboplastin time and the prothrombin time.* These are significantly prolonged, due to the depletion of clotting factors.

3 *The fibrinogen concentration.* This can be estimated either on the basis of the time taken for a diluted sample of plasma to clot in the presence of high concentrations of thrombin (Clauss method) or by immunological or clinical methods.

4 *The thrombin time.* When the fibrinogen concentration is normal, estimation of the thrombin time is a useful indication of the presence of excessive amounts of FDP. The thrombin time is determined by adding low concentrations of thrombin to citrated plasma and measuring the time for the appearance of a clot. In the presence of FDP, the thrombin time is prolonged due to inhibition of fibrin polymerization.

5 *Estimation of FDP.* The presence of FDP can be detected by a rapid immunological test in which latex particles coated with antibody directed against fibrinogen are agglutinated by FDP present in serum.

Treatment

Since the activation of the clotting system is the primary initiating stimulus and fibrinolysis is mainly a secondary phenomenon, treatment is aimed at preventing further coagulation by removal of the initiating cause (e.g. when it occurs in obstetric practice, rapid and non-traumatic vaginal delivery stops the clotting process). Whilst the initiating cause is being dealt with, patients with acute DIC should be supported with transfusions of blood, fresh-frozen plasma and platelet concentrates in order to restore blood volume and replace clotting factors and platelets.

Anticoagulant drugs

The two most frequently used anticoagulant drugs are heparin (Hirsh 1991) and warfarin (BCSH 1990a). Intravenous heparin is used in patients with deep vein thrombosis (DVT) or pulmonary embolism (PE) and is followed by warfarin therapy to reduce the risk of recurrence. The same combination is used in acute anterior transmural myocardial infarction to decrease the possibility of systemic embolism. Subcutaneous heparin is used to reduce the risk of DVT and PE in patients undergoing surgery (especially hip surgery) and in patients with acute myocardial infarction. Heparin does not cross the placenta and is therefore the preferred drug when anticoagulation is required during pregnancy. The oral anticoagulant warfarin is administered usually for 3–6 months to patients with DVT or PE or after insertion of xenograft mitral heart valves or coronary by-pass surgery. Life-long warfarin therapy is indicated in patients with recurrent venous thrombosis, with rheumatic mitral valve disease complicated by embolism or atrial fibrillation, and with prosthetic heart valves. It is considered in patients with congenital deficiencies of antithrombin III, protein C or protein S, and for patients with the lupus anticoagulant.

HEPARIN

Standard unfractionated heparin is an acidic mucopolysaccharide (average molecular weight 1.5×10^4 daltons) which has to be administered intravenously or subcutaneously. When administered intravenously, it's biological half-life is 1 hour. Heparin potentiates the action of antithrombin III, a molecule which inactivates the activated serine protease coagulation factors, thrombin (IIa), IXa, Xa and XIa; the greatest effect is on IIa. Low molecular weight heparin (average molecular weight 4–5 x 10^3 daltons) is used subcutaneously; it inactivates Xa to a greater extent than IIa and has a longer biological half-life.

For the treatment of thrombosis or embolism, standard heparin is best administered as a bolus of 5000 units (70 units/kg) intravenously, followed by a continuous intravenous infusion of 15–25 units/kg/hour. Treatment is monitored by performing the activated partial thromboplastin time, the heparin dosage being altered so as to maintain the APTT at 1.5–2.5 times the normal value. When a patient on heparin is started on warfarin, there should be a minimum overlap period of 3 days and the heparin should be stopped only when a full warfarin effect is achieved.

Either standard or low molecular weight heparin is administered subcutaneously to prevent venous thrombosis in patients subjected to surgery or in patients with myocardial infarction or when long-term heparin therapy is required. The dosage of standard heparin for prevention of post-operative thrombosis is 5000 units subcutaneously pre-operatively followed by 5000 units subcutaneously 12 hourly for 7 days or until the patient is fully mobile. Low molecular weight heparin is administered once daily.

Haemorrhage due to overdosage is managed by stopping the heparin and, if necessary, by giving protamine sulphate intravenously. Side-effects include thrombocytopenia (due to an effect of heparin on platelet function or due to anti-heparin antibodies), osteoporosis (following long-term use), alopecia and hypersensitivity reactions.

WARFARIN SODIUM

This is a coumarin derivative that is administered orally, once a day. As has already been mentioned, it is a vitamin K antagonist and interferes with the carboxylation and hence with the functional activity of factors II, VII, IX, X, protein C and protein S. After the first dose, clotting factor activity is reduced in the order VII, IX, X and II (i.e. the factor with the shortest half-life is reduced fastest and the longest half-life most slowly).

It is customary to prescribe 10 mg warfarin on the first day and to determine the prothrombin ratio (the ratio of the patient's prothrombin time to the mean normal prothrombin time) and the International Normalized Ratio or INR (i.e. the prothrombin ratio standardized by correcting for the sensitivity of the thromboplastin used) 16 hours later. Subsequent doses are based on the INR. The therapeutic ranges of INR commonly recommended are 2–3 for a first DVT or PE, transient ischaemic attacks, arterial disease, arterial grafts and to prevent systemic embolism in patients with atrial fibrillation, mitral valve disease, myocardial infarction or tissue heart valves. A higher range of 3–4 is used for recurrent DVT or PE, recurrent systemic embolism and for patients with prosthetic heart valves.

There are many possible causes for loss of control of warfarin therapy. These include the simultaneous use of drugs that, decrease absorption of vitamin K (e.g. antibiotics or laxatives), reduce binding of warfarin to albumin (e.g. phenylbutazone) or inhibit hepatic microsomal degradation (e.g. cimetidene). Bleeding is controlled by stopping the warfarin, and if serious, also by infusing fresh-frozen plasma and by administering vitamin K (2–5 mg i.v.). Vitamin K therapy is followed by a period of resistance to warfarin.

Warfarin crosses the placenta and may cause developmental abnormalities such a chondrodysplasia, microcephaly and blindness. It is therefore contraindicated in the first trimester of pregnancy. It should also not be administered during the last few weeks of pregnancy because of its anticoagulant effect on the fetus and the consequent risk of fetal or placental haemorrhage.

Investigation of a patient with abnormal bleeding

A most important step in the diagnostic process is the taking of a good history from the patient (Biggs 1968). The physician should ask, amongst others, the following questions: Has the patient ever bled excessively in the past and have any relatives bled excessively? More specifically, has the patient had tonsillectomy, major abdominal or orthopaedic surgery or dental extractions in the past, and if so was there any abnormal bleeding? The excellent paper of Ingram (1977) should be consulted for a more detailed discussion of the taking of the patient's own, and family history. The relationship between the type of bleeding and the nature of the haemostatic defect has been discussed earlier (p. 203).

The screening tests that are useful in investigating a patient who gives a history of excessive bleeding are the following:

1   blood count, including a platelet count;
2   examination of a blood film;
3   bleeding time;
4   prothrombin time;
5   activated partial thromboplastin time;
6   thrombin time;
7   fibrinogen assay, and
8   euglobulin clot lysis time (a global test for fibrinolysis).

If any of these tests is found to be abnormal, further specialized tests may be necessary.

Natural anticoagulant mechanisms and the pre-thrombotic state (thrombophilia)

There are natural anticoagulant mechanisms in the plasma which prevent localized fibrin formation from becoming widespread. The most important molecules involved in these mechanisms are antithrombin III, protein C and protein S, all of which are produced in the liver. Inherited or acquired abnormalities of these inhibitors of coagulation may lead to a pre-thrombotic state (thrombophilia) (BCSH 1990b). This section summarizes the essential information relating to: (a) the congenital deficiency of these factors; (b) a pre-thrombotic state due to the presence of a specific mutation in factor V; and (c) one acquired pre-thrombotic state known as the lupus anticoagulant syndrome.

ANTITHROMBIN III

As its name implies, this is mainly an inhibitor of thrombin, but it also inhibits factors IXa, Xa and XIa; its action is markedly potentiated by heparin (Beresford 1988). Normally some antithrombin III (AT III) becomes activated by binding to endothelial-cell-associated heparan sulphate and thus prevents thrombus formation on the endothelium. Congenital AT III deficiency is inherited as an autosomal dominant character; its prevalence is about 1 in 1500. Heterozygotes (whose AT III concentrations are 40–50% of normal) may suffer from recurrent deep vein thrombosis, mesenteric vein thrombosis and pulmonary embolism; the first thrombotic event usually occurs between the ages of 15 and 50 years. Homozygotes present in childhood with severe venous or arterial thrombosis or both.

PROTEIN C AND PROTEIN S

Two other inhibitors of coagulation are the vitamin-K-dependent substances protein C and protein S (BCSH 1990b). Protein C becomes activated when it reacts with thrombin bound to thrombomodulin, a protein of the endothelial cell membrane. Activated protein C is a serine protease and degrades factors Va and VIIIa; it also promotes fibrinolysis by inactivating PAI-1 (p. 217). Protein S potentiates the effects of activated protein C.

Some individuals have a hereditary deficiency of protein C, with about 50% of normal levels; these are heterozygotes for a mutation affecting the protein C gene and in one study were found with a prevalence of about 1 per 250. A proportion of such heterozygotes displays the clinical picture seen in inherited AT III deficiency but in addition are particularly prone to develop superficial thrombophlebitis, cerebral vein thrombosis and coumarin-induced skin necrosis. Homozygotes for the mutant gene are rare, and those who have virtually no protein C present with purpura fulminans or extensive thrombosis of visceral veins in the neonatal period.

Some heterozygotes for protein S deficiency suffer from recurrent venous thromboembolism. Homozygotes are severely affected and suffer from purpura fulminans in the neonatal period.

The incidence of protein C deficiency in children and adults below the age of 45 years with recurrent venous thrombosis is about 5% and the incidence of protein S deficiency in this group is similar.

Resistance to activated protein C (APC)

An abnormality inherited as an autosomal dominant character confers resistance to the anticoagulant effects of APC and is associated with a familial tendency to deep vein thrombosis. Recently, this abnormality has been shown to be a specific mutant factor Va (Arg^{506}→Gln) which is poorly degraded by APC (Zöller et al. 1994). APC resistance may be five to ten times more common than deficiencies of antithrombin III, protein C or protein S; it is found in 5% of healthy subjects (Koster et al. 1993). Some homozygotes for the factor V mutation suffer from myocardial infarction at an early age.

Lupus anticoagulant syndrome

The antiphospholipid antibody syndrome, also known as the lupus anti-coagulant syndrome or the anticardiolipin syndrome, is defined by the presence of antiphospholipid antibodies which prolong coagulation tests, such as the activated partial thromboplastin time, which depend on phospholipid. Features of this syndrome may include thrombocytopenia, recurrent arterial or venous thromboses and recurrent abortions. Antiphospholipid antibodies are found in some patients with SLE or other autoimmune disorders as well as in individuals with no other evidence of an immunological abnormality. The mechanisms underlying the throm-botic tendency in patients with antiphospholipid antibodies are uncer-tain. Patients who have suffered a thrombotic event are treated long term with anti-platelet drugs or anticoagulants.

References

Baker W.F., Jr. (1989) Clinical aspects of disseminated intravascular coagulation: a clinicians point of view. Semin. Thromb. Hemost. **15**, 1–57.

BCSH (British Committee for Standards in Haematology) (1990a) Guidelines on oral anticoagulation. J. Clin. Pathol. **43**, 177–183.

BCSH (British Committee for Standards in Haematology) (1990b) Guidelines on the investigation and management of thrombophilia. J. Clin. Pathol. **43**, 703–709.

Beresford C.H. (1988) Antithrombin III deficiency. Blood Rev. **2**, 239–250.

Bick R.L. (1994) Disseminated intravascular coagulation. Objective criteria for diagnosis and management. Med. Clin. North Am. **78**, 511–543.

Biggs R. (1968) The detection of defects in blood coagulation. Br. J. Haematol. **15**, 115–117.

Biggs R., Douglas A.S., MacFarlane R.G., Dacie J.V., Pitney W.R., Merskey C., O'Brien J.R. (1952) Christmas disease: a condition previously mistaken for haemophilia. Br. Med. J. **2**, 1378–1382.

Doan C.A., Bouroncle B.A., Wiseman B.K. (1960) Idiopathic and secondary thrombo-cytopenic purpura: clinical study and evaluation of 381 cases over a period of 28 years. Ann. Int. Med. **53**, 861–876.

Eyster M.E., Gill F.M., Blatt P.M., Hilgartner M.W., Ballard J.O., Kinney T.R. et al. (1978) Central nervous system bleeding in haemophiliacs. Blood **51**, 1179–1188.

Harker L. A., Slichter S. J. (1972) The bleeding time as a screening test for evaluation of platelet function. N. Engl. J. Med. **287**, 155–159.

Hirsh J. (1991) Heparin. N. Engl. J. Med. **324**, 1565–1574.

Hoyer L.W. (1994) Hemophilia A. N. Engl. J. Med. **330**, 38–47.

Imbach P.A. (1994) Harmful and beneficial antibodies in immune thrombocytopenic purpura. Clin. Exp. Immunol. **97**, Suppl. 1, 25–30.

Ingram G.I.C. (1977) Investigation of a long-standing bleeding tendency. Br. Med. Bull. **33**, 261–264.

Karpatkin S. (1980) Autoimmune thrombocytopenic purpura. Blood. **56**, 329–343.

Kazazian H.H., Jr. (1993) The molecular basis of hemophilia A and the present status of carrier and antenatal diagnosis of the disease. Thromb. Haemost. **70**, 60–62.

Kirchner J.T. (1992) Acute and chronic immune thrombocytopenic purpura. Disorders that differ in more than duration. Postgrad. Med. **92**, 112–118, 125–126.

Koster T., Rosendaal F.R., de Ronde H., Briët E., Vandenbroucke J.P., Berting R.M. (1993) Venous thrombosis due to poor anticoagulant response to activated protein C: Leiden thrombophilia study. Lancet **342**, 1503–1506.

Lethagen S. (1993) von Willebrand's disease. Pathogenesis and clinical aspects. Crit. Rev. Oncol. Hematol. **15**, 1–11.

MacFarlane R.G. (1964) An enzyme cascade in the blood-clotting mechanism, and its function as a biochemical amplifier. Nature **202**, 498.

MacFarlane R.G. (1969) The blood clotting mechanism. The development of a theory of blood coagulation. Proc. R. Soc. B. **173**, 261–268.

Muller-Berghaus G. (1989) Pathophysiologic and biochemical events in disseminated intravascular coagulation: dysregulation of procoagulant and anticoagulant pathways. Semin. Thromb. Hemost. **15**, 58–87.

Rick M.E. (1994) Diagnosis and management of von Willebrand's syndrome. Med. Clin. North Am. **78**, 609–623.

Rizza C.R. (1977) Clinical management of haemophilia. Br. Med. Bull. **33**, 225–230.

Rizza C.R., Spooner R.J.D. (1977) Home treatment of haemophilia and Christmas disease: five years experience. Br. J. Haematol. **37**, 53–66.

Rodeghiero F., Castaman G., Mannucci P.M. (1991) Clinical indications for desmopressin (DDAVP) in congenital and acquired von Willebrand's disease. Blood Rev. **5**, 153–161.

Zöller B., Svensson P., He X., Dahlback B. (1994) Identification of the same factor V gene mutation in 47 out of 50 thrombosis-prone families with inherited resistance to activated protein C. J. Clin. Invest. **94**, 2521–2524.

Reviews

Bloom A.L., Forbes C.D., Thomas D.F., Tuddenham E.G.D. (eds.) (1994) Haemostasis and Thrombosis, 3rd edn, Vols 1 & 2. Churchill Livingstone, Edinburgh.

Colman R.W., Rao A.K. (eds.) (1990) Platelets in health and disease. Hematol./Oncol. Clin. North Am. **4**, 1–313.

Furie B., Furie B.C. (1990) Molecular basis of haemophilia. Sem. Hematol. **27**, 270–285.

Hirsh J. (ed.) (1990) Anti-thrombotic therapy. Clin. Haematol. **3**, 483–830.

Lee C.A. (1992) Coagulation factor replacement therapy. In: Hoffbrand A.V., Brenner M.K. (eds.) Recent Advances in Haematology, Vol 6, pp. 73–88. Churchill Livingstone, Edinburgh.

Meade T.W. (1994) Thrombophilia. Baillière's Clinical Haematology. International Practice and Research, Vol 7/No 3. Baillière Tindall, London.

Page C.P. (ed.) (1991) *The Platelet in Health and Disease*. Blackwell Scientific Publications, Oxford.

Ratnoff O.D., Forbes C.D. (1991) *Disorders of Hemostasis*, 2nd edn. W.B. Saunders, Philadelphia.

Tuddenham E.G.D. (ed.) (1991) The molecular biology of coagulation. *Clin. Haematol.* **2**, 787–1042.

Warnock L.J. (1991) The application of molecular biology techniques to haemostasis and thrombosis. *Blood Coagul. Fibrinolysis* **2**, 529–538.

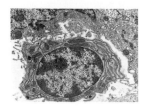

Blood Transfusion and Haemolytic Disease of the Newborn

Objectives in learning

1 To know about the inheritance of the ABO system, and the type and distribution of associated antibodies.

2 To know the distribution and mode of inheritance of the D antigen of the Rh system.

3 To know the principles involved in the selection of donor blood of suitable ABO and Rh groups for a recipient, and the principles of the cross-match, including the antiglobulin test.

4 To know the hazards of blood transfusion (incompatible blood, pyrogenic and allergic reactions, bacterial infection, citrate toxicity and transmission of disease) and of massive blood transfusion.

5 To know how to investigate a patient suspected of receiving an incompatible transfusion.

6 To know the basis of blood fractionation and the rationale for the use of specific blood products, including red cells, platelet concentrates, fresh-frozen plasma (FFP) and various factor concentrates.

7 To understand the principles of requesting blood for routine surgical procedures.

8 To know the pathogenesis, clinical features and the principles underlying the treatment and prevention of haemolytic disease of the newborn (HDN) due to anti-D.

9 To know the principles of antenatal care concerned with predicting both the presence and severity of HDN due to anti-D.

10 To know the differences between HDN due to anti-D and that due to anti-A and anti-B.

Blood transfusion

One of the main problems in the transfusion of blood is the avoidance of immunological reactions resulting from the differences in the chemical constituents of the red cells between donor and recipient. Blood groups have arisen because mutations have occurred in the genes controlling the surface constituents of the red cells. These alterations in the surface structures have not usually affected the function of the red cell, but when the red cells of a donor are transfused into a recipient who lacks these surface structures, the recipient treats them as foreign substances and produces antibodies against them. There are 22 major sites on the chromosomes where there are genes responsible for red-cell surface constituents, and each of these sites is responsible for a different blood-group system. Although all the systems have given rise to transfusion difficulties (and in fact this is how many have been recognized), only two, the ABO and Rh systems, are of major importance.

ABO SYSTEM

The ABO system (Contreras 1992) has three allelic genes, A, B and O. The first two genes are responsible for converting a basic substance, H, present in every red cell, into A or B substances, thus converting the cells into groups A or B. The O gene has no known effect on the H substance, so that group O red cells simply contain H substance. H substance is a carbohydrate chain combined to lipid or protein in the red-cell membrane. A terminal sugar molecule is attached to this chain which determines the antigenic specificity, N-acetylgalactosamine in the case of A antigen, and galactose in the case of B antigen. The A and B genes each code for the two different enzymes (glycosyltransferases) which attach these terminal groups. The O gene has no recognized product. The three allelomorphic genes combine in pairs to give six possible genotypes, AA, AO, BB, BO, AB and OO.

In determining the blood group of a person, it is necessary to distinguish between genotype and phenotype. Genotype refers to the specific genes that the person carries, whereas the phenotype refers to the observed characteristics, that is, the agglutination reactions brought about by the appropriate antibodies. Determination of the ABO blood group of a person is carried out using only two antibodies, anti-A and anti-B, through agglutination reactions. Genotypes can only be determined by family studies, e.g. the genotype AO and AA cannot be distinguished by agglutinating antibodies and both of these genotypes will be classified as the phenotype A. Thus, only four phenotypes are distinguished, namely A, B, AB and O. As the phenotype A includes the genotypes AA and AO, it follows that a mating between two people of phenotype A can produce a child of group O, if both parents are genotypically AO. The same principle holds for the phenotype B.

The frequency of the ABO groups differs in different populations; in the UK it is approximately: group O, 46%; A, 42%; B, 9%; and AB, 3%.

Substances with antigenic properties closely similar to those of A and B are widely distributed in nature and are found in many animals and bacteria. Absorption of these substances from the gut is presumed to give rise to the production of anti-A and anti-B in the plasma of those who do not possess the substances on their red cells. Because of the presence of these antibodies it is necessary to transfuse blood with the same ABO group as that of the recipient. People of group O were at one time known as 'universal donors'. However, this is a dangerous concept, because group O people have anti-A and anti-B in their plasma, and in a small number of people these antibodies may be very potent so that a unit of group O blood may contain sufficient anti-A or anti-B to react with the recipient's cells and bring about their destruction.

Rh SYSTEM

The Rh system derives its name from the findings of K. Landsteiner and A.S. Wiener (1940) that the antibody produced in rabbits by the injection of red cells from the Rhesus monkey would agglutinate the red cells of 85% of humans (Rh-positive) but not of the remaining 15% (Rh-negative). It was quickly disovered that a similar antibody could also be found in the plasma of humans after blood transfusion, and in the plasma of mothers who had given birth to a child with HDN. Several other antibodies were found in humans which were clearly recognizing antigens within the Rh system and in 1943, R.A. Fisher put forward the theory that there are three allelomorphic pairs of genes within the Rh system, C and c, D and d, E and e. It was postulated that each gene was responsible for producing a different protein molecule on the surface of the red cell, termed C, c, D, d, E and e. Recent genetic analysis however has shown that the genetic structure is more complex in that there are only two genes, RHD and RHCE. The RHD gene is responsible for the production of the D protein; there is no d gene and Rh-negative people are those in whom the D gene is absent. The other gene, RHCE is responsible for the C, c, E and e antigens. There are four common alleles of this gene, namely CE, Ce, cE and ce. Each of these genes gives rise to both the C/c and E/e proteins by a process of differential translation e.g. the CE allele gives rise to both the C and E proteins. Thus, individuals carrying the CE and ce genes (one on each chromosome) will have C, E, c and e proteins on the surface of their red cells.

People who were labelled as Rh-positive on the old nomenclature have the D antigen on their red cells. Thus, people who are either homozygous DD, or heterozygous Dd, are Rh-positive. Despite the non-existence of d, it is convenient to retain the symbol d and the genotype dd for Rh-negative people to indicate the absence of D. The two genes RHD and RHCE are on chromosome 1 and lie very close together since no crossing-over has ever been found. Thus they are always inherited as a specific combination, the three most common being *DCe*, *dce* and *DcE*. As one of the chromosomes in each chromosome pair is derived from the father and one from the mother, the final genotype might be *DCe/dce*, which is the commonest combination. Rh-negative blood-transfusion donors are always *dce/dce*. Differentiation of people into the Rh-positive and Rh-negative groups is carried out only with anti-D antibody. Use of an antibody of only one specificity means that homozygous *DD* people cannot be differentiated from heterozygous *Dd* people. However, since all the genes of the Rh system are inherited in specific combinations, determination of the presence or absence of the other antigens (C, c, E and e), especially when combined with family studies, can almost always differentiate *DD* from *Dd*. This assessment is sometimes required to determine whether an Rh-negative mother who has anti-D in her plasma can conceive an Rh-negative child by an Rh-positive father; this can only happen if the father is *Dd*.

Clinically, only the D antigen and anti-D are important. The reason for this is that the D antigen is a much more potent antigen than C, c, E or e. Thus, an Rh-negative person (i.e. *dce/dce*) has over 50% chance of developing anti-D after the transfusion of one unit of Rh-positive blood, whereas the 'c' antigen will only provoke anti-c production in 2% of people lacking this antigen (Mollison *et al.* 1993). It is thus important that Rh-negative people receive Rh-negative blood. On the other hand, the risk of immunization after giving Rh-negative blood (*dce/dce*) to an Rh-positive person who lacks the 'c' antigen (for instance whose genotype is *DCe/DCe*) is very small.

OTHER BLOOD-GROUP SYSTEMS

Other blood-group antibodies, which are sometimes a problem during blood transfusion, include the following: anti-K (Kell system), anti-Fy^a (Duffy system), anti-Jk^a (Kidd system) and anti-S (part of the MNSs blood group system). Unless an antibody against one of the antigens in these systems is present in the recipient, there is no need to take these groups into account in selecting donor blood. The chief reason for this is that these antigens are also 'poor' antigens. Thus, compared to the D antigen, their relative potency in stimulating antibody production is 10–1000 times less.

COMPATIBILITY

The purpose of cross-matching blood before transfusion is to ensure that there is no antibody present in the recipient's plasma which will react with any antigen on the donor's cells. The basic technique for detecting the antibody, i.e. agglutination of the red cells by antibody, has remained unchanged for over one hundred years. Agglutination was first observed in 1869 by A. Creite in Göttingen when he found that the serum of one animal would agglutinate red cells of another species; the fact that the agglutinating agents were antibodies was not discovered until 1890.

Unfortunately, many red-cell antibodies are unable to bring about agglutination without additional help, such as proteolytic treatment of the red cells or the use of an antiglobulin reagent (see below). The ability of antibodies to agglutinate untreated red cells depends partly on the molecular structure of the antibody. IgM antibodies (molecular weight 9×10^5 daltons) are large and readily span between adjacent red cells and thus can bring about agglutination. By contrast, the smaller IgG antibodies (1.6×10^5 daltons), which are far more common than IgM, do not usually agglutinate, the main exception being IgG anti-A and -B.

The antiglobulin test

The antiglobulin test was first discovered by C. Moreschi in 1908, but was forgotten as it had no practical significance at that time, and rediscovered by R.R.A. Coombs, A.E. Mourant and R.R. Race in 1945. The basic constituent of an antiglobulin serum is anti-human IgG and is obtained by injecting human IgG into animals. Being bivalent, anti-IgG is able to bring about agglutination of IgG-coated red cells by linking IgG molecules on one red cell with those on an adjacent red cell and thus holding the cells together as agglutinates.

The antiglobulin test can be used in two ways. Firstly, it can be used to detect antibody already on the patient's cells in vivo. Red cells are washed to remove the free IgG in the plasma, which would otherwise react with and neutralize the antiglobulin. After washing, antiglobulin serum is added and agglutination takes place (the direct antiglobulin test). Secondly, the test can be used to detect the presence of antibody in serum, as in the cross-matching of blood for transfusion. In this case, serum from the patient requiring transfusion is incubated with red cells from the donor blood. Any antibody present in the recipient's serum which has specificity for antigens on the donor's cells will combine with the latter and, after washing, addition of antiglobulin serum will bring about agglutination (the indirect antiglobulin test).

Procedure for obtaining compatible blood

The ABO and Rh group of the recipient must first be determined by the addition of agglutinating anti-A and anti-B to the red cells and the grouping is checked by determining whether anti-A or anti-B is present in the recipient's serum by adding known group A and B cells; group A blood always contains anti-B in the plasma, group B blood has anti-A and group O has anti-A and anti-B. The Rh group is determined using an agglutinating IgM anti-D or by using IgG anti-D combined with the antiglobulin test.

Donor blood of the appropriate ABO and Rh group is then selected but before this can be transfused, cross-matching must be carried out, partly to ensure that there have been no errors in the determination of the ABO group of the donor and recipient, and partly to ensure that no other antibodies are present in the recipient which react with the donor's red cells. A search is made for both agglutinating and non-agglutinating antibodies, the latter with the antiglobulin test.

In most transfusion laboratories, it is now usual for the sera of all recipients to be screened for the presence of antibodies such as anti-K (Kell), anti-Fy^a (Duffy) and anti-Jk^a (Kidd), using a panel of red cells of known phenotype, whenever time permits. If screening is not carried out, these antibodies will be discovered in the final stages of a cross-matching procedure, using the antiglobulin test.

Rh-negative donor blood is not always available for Rh-negative recipients and the question arises whether it is safe to give Rh-positive blood. Rh-negative males, especially elderly males, may receive Rh-positive blood provided care is taken to search for anti-D if subsequent transfusions of Rh-positive blood are given. In women past the menopause the procedure is less safe because there is always the possibility, admittedly small, that they may have received a primary stimulus with D antigen from an Rh-positive fetus and the anti-D in the plasma may be below a detectable level. Transfusion of Rh-positive blood would then provoke a secondary response of anti-D production leading to a delayed transfusion reaction after a few days. Rh-positive blood must never be given to Rh-negative girls or Rh-negative women of child-bearing age for fear of stimulating anti-D production and thus of producing HDN in a subsequent pregnancy.

Ensuring that the patient receives the correct blood

Incompatible transfusions are only rarely due to mismatching of blood in the laboratory. Responsibility for giving the wrong blood usually lies with the person who takes the sample of the recipient's blood for cross-matching or with the person who sets up the transfusion. When taking blood for cross-matching, great care should be taken that this is correctly labelled with the patients' name and hospital number and the label should be signed by the person who takes the sample. The person who sets up the transfusion is responsible for ensuring that the patient's name and hospital number on the compatibility label of the unit of blood apply to the patient who is being transfused and also that the serial number on the compatibility label is the same as the serial number of the bag of blood. It must be emphasized that the commonest cause of incompatible transfusions is the carelessness of those responsible for setting up the transfusions. The patient must be particularly closely observed during the first 5 minutes and reviewed 20 minutes following the start of the transfusion, to detect any evidence of a reaction due to incompatible or infected blood. This precaution is important, since symptoms of an incompatible transfusion usually appear within this time and, if the transfusion is stopped at an early stage, the chance of a fatal outcome is reduced.

DONOR BLOOD

Donor blood (approximately 450 ml) is mixed with citrate-phosphate-dextrose containing adenine (CPD-adenine), a solution found empirically to give good preservation of the blood. If the blood is stored at 4°C, 80% of the cells are still viable after 28 days, the remaining 20% being removed from the circulation by the reticuloendothelial system within a few hours of transfusion. After 35 days of storage, the percentage of viable cells falls off fairly rapidly, so that the blood is not used after this period of time. Stored blood has reduced levels of red cell 2,3-DPG (p. 2) but levels return to at least 50% of normal within 24 hours of transfusion. When plasma is removed from CPD-adenine blood to prepare fresh-frozen plasma or plasma products or platelet and granulocyte concentrates, the red cells may be transfused after storage for up to 35 days either in CPD-adenine or, if all the plasma is removed, in a solution containing saline, adenine, glucose and mannitol (SAG-M).

TRANSFUSION IN ACUTE HAEMORRHAGE AND CHRONIC ANAEMIAS

Patients with acute haemorrhage (i.e. loss of red cells and plasma) should be transfused with whole blood or with red cells suspended in SAG-M. If more than ten units of stored blood have to be transfused within 24 hours (massive transfusion), patients may need platelet transfusions and fresh-frozen plasma (p. 250). Plasma-reduced blood with a packed cell volume (PCV) of about 65% or concentrated red cells in SAG-M should be used when patients with a severe chronic anaemia have to be transfused, as such patients have an increased plasma volume and are prone to develop circulatory overload (p. 246). Leucocyte-poor blood, usually prepared by filtering plasma-reduced blood, is used in patients on a long-term blood transfusion programme or in those who have repeated febrile transfusion reactions due to white cell antibodies.

Hazards of blood transfusion

Since the appearance of AIDS, the attitude of the general public to blood transfusion has completely changed and there is now a demand for transfusion without risks, although this can never be achieved (Zuck 1987). The hazards of transfusion have to be evaluated in terms of risk analysis and the concept of 'risk tolerance' is the most important aspect. The term 'risk tolerance' was first introduced in a report in relation to nuclear power in the UK but is equally applicable to transfusion. To quote this report 'Tolerability does not mean acceptability. It refers to the willingness to live with risks to secure benefits and in the confidence that it is being properly controlled. To tolerate a risk means that we do not regard it as negligible or something that we might ignore, but rather as something we need to keep under review and to reduce still further if and as we can' (Layfield 1987).

The unfavourable reactions to transfusion are either immediate or delayed; immediate reactions are usually due to pyrogens, allergens, bacteria, circulatory overloading or incompatible blood; delayed reactions are due to the transmission of disease, usually of viral origin.

HAEMOLYTIC REACTIONS DUE TO INCOMPATIBLE RED CELLS

The symptoms that are found after a transfusion of incompatible blood depend on whether the transfused cells suffer intravascular lysis or whether they are phagocytosed by the reticuloendothelial system and subjected to extravascular lysis. Intravascular lysis leads to haemoglobinaemia and haemoglobinuria and is almost always due to the action of anti-A or anti-B which bring about lysis in conjunction with the complement system. Symptoms may appear from a few minutes to several hours after beginning to transfuse ABO incompatible blood and may include restlessness, anxiety, fever, chills, flushing of the face, pain in the lumbar region and chest, vomiting and diarrhoea. If the reaction is severe, there is circulatory collapse. These effects result from the release into the plasma of the complement fragments C3a, C4a and C5a which cause contraction of smooth muscle and degranulation of mast cells. Sometimes, extensive haemorrhage may occur due to DIC (p. 228) as a consequence of the release of tissue thromboplastin from lysed red cells and hypoxic tissue. There is also about a 10% chance of developing oliguria or anuria; this is probably a consequence of hypotension and DIC.

The immediate treatment of a mismatched transfusion is to promote diuresis with frusemide. When deaths do occur, they are usually the result either of severe DIC or of renal failure. The overall mortality following ABO incompatibility is probably of the order of 10%. In a survey involving 130 000 recipients of blood, four deaths from 40 incompatible transfusions were reported (Wallace 1977).

When blood transfusion is followed by extravascular destruction of red cells, there are usually only chills and fever occurring one or more hours after the start of the transfusion. The most common antibody causing extravascular destruction is anti-D. This type of incompatibility is almost never followed by renal failure.

Another type of incompatibility is the delayed haemolytic transfusion reaction. This occurs when a recipient has been previously immunized by transfusion or pregnancy but in whom the antibody in the plasma has become too weak to be identified. Following the transfusion, a secondary immunological response takes place and the antibody titre rapidly rises, bringing about haemolysis, usually about seven days later. Typically, the patient develops anaemia, fever, jaundice and sometimes haemoglobinuria. The incidence of this type of reaction may be as high as 1 per 4000 recipients (Pineda et al. 1978).

PYREXIA DUE TO PYROGENS AND LEUCOCYTE ANTIBODIES

Febrile reactions occur during 0.5–1% of transfusions. Reactions due to the presence of pyrogens (soluble bacterial polysaccharides) in the anticoagulant are now extremely uncommon. Most febrile reactions are caused by the presence in the recipient of anti-HLA antibodies or granulocyte-specific antibodies, resulting from immunization during pregnancy or previous transfusions. They usually consist of chills and fever starting 30–60 minutes after the onset of the transfusion. Such reactions can often be prevented by the administration of an antipyretic or by using leucocyte-poor red cells (p. 243). Since reactions due to pyrogens are now rare, febrile reactions should always suggest the possibility that incompatible red cells or leucocytes have been transfused.

IMMEDIATE-TYPE HYPERSENSITIVITY

Hypersensitivity reactions may occur soon after the transfusion of blood or plasma. The antibodies involved are often unknown but some severe reactions are caused by antibodies against IgA present in recipients who lack IgA and who have previously become sensitized to this immunoglobulin. In mild cases, the only manifestation may be urticarial wheals, erythema, maculopapular rash or periorbital oedema. In the more severe reactions, hypotension may occur; bronchial spasm and laryngeal oedema are rare. Mild reactions probably occur in about 1–3%

of transfusions and can be treated with antihistamines. Severe reactions are very infrequent (1 : 20 000) and these require the administration of hydrocortisone and adrenaline.

BACTERIAL CONTAMINATION

Transfusion of infected blood is rare, but when it does occur is frequently lethal. Bacterial contamination can occur at several points (contaminated blood bags, donor venepuncture or at the time of transfusion). Bacteria that have been implicated are usually normal skin flora or other ubiquitous organisms. Skin contaminants entering donor blood are usually staphylococci but these are killed off during storage and are only rarely found after 3 weeks. Occasionally, however, Gram-negative bacteria enter donor blood and these will grow slowly at 4°C (doubling time about 8 hours). In 2–3 weeks at 4°C, growth can be sufficient to cause a lethal reaction. The growth rate of these bacteria is considerably speeded up if the blood is kept at room temperature and the risks of transfusing infected blood can thus be minimized by keeping blood at 4°C until the moment of transfusion. The chief signs of transfusion of infected blood are the rapid onset of pyrexia and circulatory collapse. Haemorrhage due to disseminated intravascular coagulation may occur.

CIRCULATORY OVERLOAD

Circulatory overload with consequent cardiac failure can easily be brought about by the too rapid transfusion of blood, especially in the elderly and in those who have been severely anaemic for some time. The first signs are dyspnoea, a dry cough, crepitations at the lung bases and a rise in jugular venous pressure. The transfusion must be stopped and venesection may be necessary. The risk of overload can be minimized in patients with severe anaemia by administering frusemide, giving concentrated red cells (p. 243) and restricting the rate of transfusion to 1 ml/kg body weight/hour. If the patient is only mildy anaemic and has normal cardiac function, 1 litre can be safely transfused over a 5 hour period. This is about one drop per second with the standard giving sets.

CITRATE TOXICITY

Citrate toxicity may develop and can cause death if large volumes of stored blood have to be given very rapidly. It is due to the reduction in ionized calcium in the patient's plasma. The signs are gross skeletal muscle tremors and prolongation of the QT interval in the ECG. If more than 2 litres are given every 20 minutes then each litre should be accompanied by 1 g of calcium gluconate.

TRANSMISSION OF DISEASE

The most important infective agents that may be transmitted are the hepatits B and C viruses and the human immunodeficiency viruses (Leikola 1993).

Post-transfusion hepatitis

Viruses known to cause post-transfusion hepatitis include the hepatitis viruses A, B and C, cytomegalovirus (CMV) and the Epstein–Barr virus (EBV). The hepatitis A, B and C viruses are endemic in the global population; hepatitis A is transmitted by the faeco-oral route, hepatitis B and C by sexual intercourse and by syringes and needles contaminated with blood. Transmission by transfusion and the use of blood products accounts for only about 1–2% of all clinical cases of hepatitis (Osmon et al. 1987)

Hepatitis A virus does not induce a chronic carrier state or chronic hepatitis and post-transfusion hepatitis A is rare. Post-transfusion hepatitis B and C are the two conditions of major concern because of the tendency for a chronic liver infection to develop in a substantial proportion of patients and, in the case of hepatitis B, a high fatality rate from fulminant hepatic failure.

Hepatitis B

Hepatitis B is a 42 nm particle containing a central core of DNA surrounded by a protein shell, which is the surface antigen; this antigen is produced in large amounts and circulates free in the plasma in the form of filaments. Its presence is readily recognized by an enzyme immunoassay and is the first viral marker to appear in the acute phase of the disease, but may disappear during convalescence before the appearance of antibodies specific for this antigen (anti-HBs). There is thus a period when neither surface antigen nor anti-HBs are present although the blood may be infective. This deficit can be overcome by detection of antibodies to the core protein (anti-HBc), which are present throughout convalescence. The use of these tests has virtually eliminated the transmission of hepatitis B. The frequency of transmission of hepatitis B in the USA was recently found to be of the order of 1 per 200 000 units transfused (Dodd 1992). In the UK, where testing for anti-HBc is not routinely performed, there are indications that the frequency of transmission may be higher.

Hepatitis C and unidentified hepatitis viruses

Post-transfusion hepatitis in which known hepatitis agents such as hepatitis A and B, CMV and EBV have been excluded used to be termed 'non A, non-B'. It is now known that a high proportion of patients with non-A, non-B hepatitis are infected with the hepatitis C organism (Choo et al. 1989), a single-stranded RNA virus. About 15% of patients with post-transfusion hepatitis are negative for both hepatitis B and C and are clearly infected with other unidentified viruses.

The hepatitis C virus (HCV) has not yet been identified by microscopy and our entire knowledge of its structure is based on recombinant gene technology applied to lymphocyte RNA; the complete sequence of the genome is now known. Antibodies have been produced specific for a number of recombinant viral proteins, and immunoassays based on them were introduced in 1989. The prevalence of anti-HCV antibodies in northern Europe and the USA is of the order of 1 in every 1000–2000 people, increasing up to 1 per 100 in areas where the virus is more common. The true incidence of viral carriers is less than this, as the presence of anti-HCV is only evidence of past infection, not of the carrier state.

One of the main problems in the detection of blood donors who are carriers is that the presence of anti-HCV is a relatively late indicator of infection, appearing on average about 3 months after innoculation but may take as long as 6–12 months to appear. Direct evidence of the presence of the virus by PCR is not yet feasible for routine donor investigation.

Clinical aspects of post-transfusion hepatitis

The onset of overt post-transfusion hepatitis varies from about 2 weeks to 6 months after the transfusion. For every case of icteric hepatitis, there are several times as many cases of anicteric hepatitis. A substantial proportion of older icteric patients with post-transfusion hepatitis B die in a fulminant phase; the mortality rate of icteric hepatitis B varies with the strain of the virus and is around 10–20%. About 10% of patients with hepatitis B also develop chronic hepatitis and some of these proceed to cirrhosis; primary hepatocellular carcinoma is also a complication.

By contrast, patients with non-A, non-B hepatitis only occasionally suffer from fulminant hepatitis (Seeff et al. 1977) but 10–50% develop a chronic hepatitis (Seeff & Hoffnagle 1977; Alter 1985) and some of these progress to cirrhosis. Hepatocellular carcinoma is also a well-established complication. Nevertheless, in a prospective study of patients with non-A, non-B hepatitis with an average follow-up period of 18 years, the incidence of death from liver disease was only slightly greater than that found in controls and was too low to alter the relative mortality rates in the two groups (Seeff et al. 1992). About one-fifth of the surviving patients still had abnormal liver function tests.

Human immunodeficiency virus (HIV)

This is an RNA virus that is transmitted sexually and through the use of syringes and needles contaminated with blood or the transfusion of blood and blood products. The first report of AIDS in three haemophiliacs appeared in 1982, and that of transfusion-associated AIDS was in an infant in 1983 and in adults in 1984. The discovery of the causative virus in 1983–1984 led to the very rapid development of assays for HIV antibody and most developed countries started screening of blood donors in 1985. The presence of HIV antibodies always seems to indicate the presence of the virus as well, that is, they do not exist as innocent markers and at least 90% of antibody-positive blood is infective. The slight risk of transfusion-transmitted HIV results from the delay between infection and the appearance of antibodies in the serum, the average delay being about 2–3 months; 95% of those infected have seroconverted by 6 months (Horsburgh et al. 1989). The risk from this latent period is reduced by appealing to donors who fall into high-risk groups to withdraw from giving blood ('self-exclusion'). At the present time, the risk of acquiring HIV in the USA as a result of the latent period is thought to be about 1 per 50 000–150 000 units; in northern Europe, it is considered to be on average about 1 per 250 000 units, but there is considerable variation in different areas depending on the incidence of the disease in the donor population. The most recent estimate for the UK is less than 1 per 1 000 000 units transfused.

The antibody screening test is an enzyme immunoassay which detects binding of both IgG and IgM antibodies to recombinant HIV antigen (both HIV1 and 2). False positives are rare but their appearance means that all positive results have to be confirmed by supplementary tests.

Factor VIII and factor IX concentrates used today carry a negligible risk of transmitting HIV. This is not only because of 'self-exclusion' and the use of anti-HIV-screened plasma for their preparation, but also because of the inactivation of any viral contamination by heat-treatment or chemical means.

Cytomegalovirus

Cytomegalovirus (CMV) is a DNA herpesvirus present in white cells. The virus is transmitted via respiratory secretions, sexually and during childbirth; the incidence of CMV antibodies varies in different parts of the world from 30 to 80% or more. As with most herpesviruses, the virus persists latently after infection. However, only a small proportion of antibody-positive blood is infective; it is thought that between 1 and 20% of all units of blood have the potential to transmit the virus (Brennan & Barbara 1993).

In normal immunocompetent people, the disease varies from a subclinical infection to the appearance of lymphadenopathy and a mild hepatitis. The main danger of CMV infection is in infants and immunocompromised patients and thus prevention of CMV infection is targeted to defined patient groups. Premature neonates of low birth weight born to mothers without anti-CMV virus are especially at risk. It has been found that 25–30% of infants with these risk factors developed the infection following transfusion and about 25% of those infected died (Adler et al. 1983). Patients receiving transplants are also at risk and the infection is the commonest cause of death following bone marrow grafting. Many transfusion centres have established panels of anti-CMV-negative donors specifically for use in these recipients.

Other diseases

Other diseases known to be transmitted by transfusion include syphilis and malaria. The prevention of transmission of syphilis is by serological testing of donors although this will not demonstrate all those infected, since it is possible to have syphilis with negative serological tests. Another factor of importance is the storage of blood at 4°C since spirochaetes do not survive for more than a few days under these conditions. Individuals who have returned from an area where malaria is endemic are not accepted as donors for 1 year, and those who were born in such an area, for 3 years. Brucellosis, babesiosis, Chagas' disease (caused by Trypanosoma cruzi), HTLV-I infection (p. 200) and parvovirus infection have also been transmitted by transfusion.

OTHER HAZARDS

Stored blood is deficient in platelets and the labile coagulation factors, V and VIII (e.g. blood stored for 5 days contains no platelets and only 30% of the normal factor VIII concentration). Therefore, massive blood transfusions lead to moderate thrombocytopenia and abnormalities in the prothrombin time and activated partial thromboplastin time. When massive blood transfusions are complicated by a haemorrhagic state, bleeding may be controlled by the administration of platelet concentrates and, if the prothrombin time is prolonged by 5 seconds or more, by fresh-frozen plasma.

As each unit of blood contains about 250 mg of iron, the administration of frequent transfusions over several years results in a marked accumulation of iron in the body (iron overload) and progressive widespread tissue damage. The iron overloading can be prevented or limited by treatment with desferrioxamine subcutaneously via a pump (see p. 93).

Procedure in the case of transfusion reactions

It is not always easy to diagnose the type of transfusion reaction by the symptoms. Allergic reactions are obvious and, if mild, only require antihistamines. Symptoms occurring within 20 minutes of starting a transfusion are often due to red-cell incompatibility or infected blood and clearly the transfusion must be stopped. It is the occurrence of rigors and fever after 30–60 minutes which causes difficulty in the diagnosis, since some of these reactions are due to bacterial pyrogens and some are due to leucocyte or red-cell incompatibility. In these patients with delayed symptoms, the transfusion should be temporarily stopped, the blood being replaced with saline, and the patient warmed. If symptoms do not rapidly disappear, the transfusion should be abandoned and the reaction investigated further. Fortunately, reactions of this type, due to incompatibility, are only rarely fatal.

INVESTIGATION OF A TRANSFUSION REACTION DUE TO INCOMPATIBILITY

There are two questions to answer after a suspected transfusion of incompatible blood: first, has destruction of red cells in fact taken place and, second, which antigen–antibody system was involved. Immediately after the transfusion has been stopped, a blood sample is obtained from the recipient and the plasma is examined for the presence of free Hb and the bilirubin concentration is estimated. A urine sample is also examined for the presence of Hb. If incompatible cells are still present in the recipient's circulation, their presence can often be detected by serological methods. Thus, the presence of group A cells in a group O patient can be detected by the addition of anti-A which will agglutinate only A cells in the sample.

The ABO and Rh group of both the recipient and donor are checked and a cross-match repeated using the serum obtained from the recipient prior to transfusion. These tests will reveal whether the incompatibility is within the ABO system or whether it involves the D antigen of the Rh system. If the ABO and Rh(D) groups are compatible, but the cross-match shows the presence of an antibody, the specificity of the antibody can be identified by further testing against a panel of red cells of known blood-group specificity. The remains of the donor blood in the pack after every transfusion should be kept at 4°C for 48 hours so that any adverse reaction can be adequately investigated.

Platelet and granulocyte concentrates

Platelet concentrates are prepared either from freshly donated units of blood or by using intermittent-flow or continuous-flow cell separators which separate platelets from blood and return the rest of the blood to the donor. They may be stored at 22°C for about 5 days. Platelet concentrates are indicated when there is clinically significant bleeding due to thrombocytopenia or a qualitative platelet defect. They should also be given prophylactically in patients with transient severe thrombocytopenia due to chemotherapy. Prior to surgery, platelet concentrates are used to obtain a platelet count between 50 and 100 $\times$ 10^9/l, depending on the nature and severity of the proposed surgical procedure. Granulocyte concentrates are prepared using cell separators and may be beneficial in patients with intractable bacterial infections associated with severe neutropenia who do not respond to antibiotics.

Haemolytic disease of the newborn

Haemolytic disease of the newborn (HDN) is a consequence of the passage of fetal red cells across the placenta resulting in the immunization of the mother to blood group antigens that she does not possess. The antibodies produced are subsequently transferred back across the placenta (only those of the IgG class are transferred) and react with the fetal red cells causing their destruction. Transplacental haemorrhage most commonly occurs at the time of labour and thus it is usually only in subsequent pregnancies that babies are affected. Before the advent of prophylactic therapy, almost all the cases (93%) were due to the anti-D of the Rh system, 6% were due to other antibodies within the Rh system and only about 1% due to antibodies in other blood group systems. Without treatment, the mortality rate of affected infants is about 20%, but the antenatal prediction of the disease, together with the introduction of treatment by exchange transfusion has considerably reduced this value. Approximately 60% of affected infants require an exchange transfusion, and in the best hands, efficient treatment results in the survival of about 95% of all those who are born alive. During the decade 1958–1968, the disease resulted in about 300–400 neonatal deaths each year in the UK and an approximately equal number were stillborn. The introduction during 1968 of prophylactic injections of anti-D into the mother immediately after labour to prevent active immunization has greatly reduced the incidence, and by the mid-1990s, only about 10–20 deaths occurred each year in the UK due to anti-D; 3–4 deaths resulted from the presence of other antibodies.

HAEMOLYTIC DISEASE DUE TO ANTI-D

The aetiology of haemolytic disease of the newborn was first elucidated by Levine and colleagues (1941). A mother who had given birth to an affected infant was transfused with her husband's blood and this was followed by a transfusion reaction. The authors correctly surmised that the mother had been immunized by a fetal antigen which had been derived from the father. The Rh blood group system was also discovered during this period and it was soon ascertained that the maternal antibody in this case was anti-Rh, now known as anti-D.

Small numbers of fetal cells can occasionally be found in the maternal circulation throughout pregnancy, especially during the third trimester, but the main transplacental passage occurs at the time of labour; the volume of the haemorrhage is usually less than 5 ml but occasionally may exceed 50 ml. There is evidence that the greater the number of fetal cells in the circulation, the greater the chance of developing antibodies (Clarke 1967, 1968). The relationship between the total amount of fetal red cells in the maternal circulation immediately after labour and the incidence of immunization of mothers 6 months later is shown in Table 12.1.

In the English population, about 17% of the women are D-negative but, before the advent of preventive therapy, only about 6% of all D-negative women became immunized to the D antigen. The reason for this is three-fold: firstly, only 83% of fathers carry the D antigen and a substantial number of these are heterozygous, hence having only a 50% chance of transmitting the *D* gene; secondly, the amount of fetal red cells crossing the placenta is often insufficient to initiate immunization; and thirdly, only about 60–70% of Rh-negative mothers are able to respond to the D-antigen by producing significant amounts of anti-D.

It is very unusual for the first-born child to be affected with HDN, the incidence being slightly less than 1% of all Rh-negative mothers who have

Table 12.1 Relationship between fetal red cells in the maternal circulation after labour and subsequent immunization of mother. (From Clarke 1968.)

INCIDENCE OF IMMUNIZATION	
Estimated number of fetal red cells (ml)	Incidence of immunization (%)
0	3.7
0.02	4.5
0.04	10.3
0.06–0.08	14.6
0.1–0.2	18.7
0.22–0.78	21.1
>0.8	23.5

no history of transfusion or abortion. The reason for this is that it is only occasionally that significant numbers of fetal red cells cross the placenta sufficiently early in pregnancy to stimulate anti-D production before the child is born.

If the fetal red cells in the mother after labour bring about a primary immunization, antibody may be found within the following 6 months. In about half the cases, however, antibody concentrations do not rise sufficiently high for anti-D to be detected at this time. During the subsequent pregnancy with an Rh-positive fetus, it only requires a few fetal red cells crossing the placenta early in pregnancy in order to provide a secondary stimulus to anti-D production, which can usually be detected by the 28th week but may not appear until the last few weeks of pregnancy.

Clinical features

There is a very great variation in the severity of the disease in the child. At one end of the scale there are infants who are not anaemic at birth and who never become jaundiced. However, the Hb concentration of these infants may fall abnormally rapidly after birth and values as low as 6 g/dl may be found up to 30 days later. All neonates with antibodies on their red cells (positive direct antiglobulin test) should therefore be followed up for a month after birth.

Moderately severely affected babies may or may not be anaemic at birth, but the rate of red-cell destruction is such that jaundice develops within a few hours. Jaundice is not seen at the time of birth since prior to this the bilirubin is excreted by placental transfer. Within 48–72 hours of birth, the plasma bilirubin may rise to 350–700 μmol/l. The rate of rise of plasma bilirubin is governed partly by the rate of red-cell destruction and partly by the degree of maturity of the bilirubin excretory mechanism, that is, on the state of development of glucuronyl transferase. As a result of the poor development of the excretory mechanism for bilirubin in many infants, it is quite common for a child with a cord Hb within the normal range (lower limit 13.5 g/dl) to become severely jaundiced. The danger associated with a high bilirubin level is kernicterus resulting from damage to the basal ganglia of the brain, with a clinical picture characterized by spasticity, arched back and death from respiratory failure. Those that survive usually have a subnormal intelligence.

Severely affected babies become so anaemic that they develop cardiac failure and are either stillborn or die shortly after birth, although those with mild cardiac failure can be resuscitated by exchange transfusion. Apart from anaemia, the characteristic feature of these children is oedema. The stillbirth rate is approximately 15% of all fetuses with haemolytic disease and death may occur from the 20th week onwards.

Management of mother and child

The ABO and Rh blood groups of all pregnant mothers are determined early in pregnancy, and all those who are Rh-negative are examined for the presence of anti-D at 12 weeks and again at 28 weeks. This latter time is chosen because if anti-D is present, this is also the optimum time for carrying out amniocentesis for the antenatal determination of the severity of the disease.

A method of predicting the severity of the disease with certainty would be very valuable since a considerable proportion of affected infants are stillborn and about half of these deaths occur after the 36th week of pregnancy, but unfortunately assessment is still very unreliable. Attempts at prediction take into account the amount of anti-D in the mother's plasma (high concentrations are associated with increased severity), the previous history of affected infants (severity runs in families) and examination of the bilirubin concentration in the amniotic fluid, which gives an indication of the extent of haemolysis. None of these is a reliable guide when taken singly, but prediction is improved when all three are considered together. Since about half the total number of stillbirths occur after the 36th week of pregnancy, induction at 36 weeks reduces the incidence of stillbirth.

When anti-D is present in the mother's plasma, cord blood is obtained at delivery and the presence of antibody on the red cells confirmed by the antiglobulin test (the strength of the reaction is no guide to severity). If the cord Hb concentration is below the normal lower limit of 13.5 g/dl, an exchange transfusion with Rh-negative blood is required. If the Hb concentration is within the normal range, the decision to give an immediate exchange transfusion rests on the cord bilirubin concentration. Some paediatricians perform an exchange transfusion if this is above 70 μmol/l but others have different criteria. Even if the cord Hb concentration is normal, death can still occur from kernicterus if the ability to excrete bilirubin is poorly developed. About half the patients with Hb concentrations within the normal range require an exchange transfusion because of a rising bilirubin concentration.

Prevention of Rh immunization

It is now possible to bring about a very considerable reduction in the incidence of Rh immunization by giving two injections of anti-D intramuscularly to an Rh-negative mother, the first at 28 weeks of pregnancy and the second within 72 hours of giving birth to an

Rh-positive child. Some centres give an additional injection at 34 weeks of pregnancy. The injected anti-D combines with the fetal red cells in the mother's circulation and brings about their destruction in the spleen. The precise mechanism by which the suppression of immunization is brought about is not known, but it is assumed that splenic destruction of fetal red cells must divert D antigen on the surface of the cells away from those sites in the immunological system where antibody production is initiated.

The effectiveness of the treatment will depend partly on the dose of anti-D that is injected after delivery. Since the anti-D acts by diverting fetal cells away from stimulating the immunological system, it is reasonable to suppose that the larger the dose, the more effective it will be, especially when the transplacental bleed is a large one. The dose of anti-D that is being used at the moment is 100–300 μg, and there is evidence that this protects against a transplacental bleed of 4–12 ml of red cells. However, it is known that 250 μg anti-D is inadequate against a bleed of 50 ml of fetal blood or more (Dudok de Wit et al. 1968) and thus larger doses of anti-D must be given when it is known that the transplacental bleed is of this order. Ideally the number of fetal red cells in the maternal circulation should be estimated using the acid-elution (Kleihauer) technique in which a dried film of maternal blood on a glass slide is dipped into a buffer solution at pH 3.5. Adult Hb is soluble in this solution but fetal Hb is not, so that subsequent counter-staining demonstrates the intact fetal red cells amongst a background of pale Hb-free maternal cells (Fig. 12.1). The dose of anti-D to be given can then be based on the extent of the feto-maternal bleed.

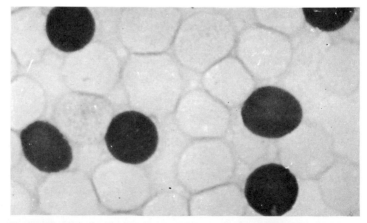

Fig. 12.1 Post-partum maternal blood film, stained by the acid elution technique of Kleihauer. The darkly-staining cells are fetal red cells present in the maternal circulation. The mother's cells have lost their haemoglobin and appear very pale.

Prophylaxis with anti-D given only after delivery reduces the incidence of HDN in the second Rh-positive child to about 0.5–1%. This figure is to be compared to an incidence of about 17% in untreated women. The failures in prevention after a single post-partum injection of anti-D are mainly due either to an inadequate dose of anti-D to cope with a large feto-maternal haemorrhage at labour (25–50 ml fetal red cells or more) or to primary immunization early in the course of the first pregnancy. The administration of anti-D both at 28 weeks and post-partum is extremely effective in preventing immunization, as has been demonstrated in the state of Manitoba where all women at risk are treated in this way. The protection rate is over 98%, with the result that perinatal deaths due to HDN have been reduced from about 20 per year to about one every 6 years (Bowman & Pollack 1983).

Anti-D should be given to all Rh-negative women having an abortion to prevent primary immunization against the D antigen. It is also possible to use anti-D to prevent primary immunization when a large amount of Rh-positive blood has been inadvertently transfused; the dose of anti-D required is of the order of 20 μg for each ml of red cells transfused.

HAEMOLYTIC DISEASE DUE TO ANTI-A AND ANTI-B

Haemolytic disease due to anti-A or anti-B is almost entirely confined to group A and B infants born to group O mothers, since it is mainly group O mothers who have anti-A and anti-B of the IgG class. ABO HDN (of all grades of severity) affects about one per 150 of all births. With the successful prophylaxis of HDN due to anti-D through the use of anti-D injections, clinically significant disease is now more frequently due to anti-A or anti-B or to antibodies other than anti-D within the Rh system, or rarely, to involvement of other blood group systems. Unlike HDN due to anti-D, ABO HDN may be seen in the first pregnancy. ABO HDN is usually very mild; still births do not occur, severe anaemia is uncommon and the child rarely requires treatment by exchange transfusion. A consistent finding is the presence of spherocytes in cord blood. In certain parts of the world, ABO HDN is even more common than in the UK. This may in part result from the high concentrations of IgG anti-A and anti-B in such populations (Lindo-Haynes 1980).

References

Adler S.P., Chaudrika T., Laurence L., Baggett J. (1983) Cytomegalovirus infections in neonates acquired by blood transfusion. *Paediatr. Infect. Dis.* **2**, 114–118.
Alter H.J. (1985) Post-transfusion hepatitis: clinical features, risk and donor testing. In: Dodd R.Y., Barker L.F. (eds.) *Infection Immunity and Blood Transfusion*, pp. 47–61. A.R. Liss, New York.

258   Chapter 12:   Blood Transfusion / HDN

Bowman J.M., Pollack J. (1983) Rh immunization in Manitoba: progress in prevention and management. *Can. Med. Assoc. J.* **129**, 343–345.

Brennan M.T., Barbara J.A.J. (1993) Transfusion-transmitted disease. *Curr. Opin. Hematol.* **1A**, 320–329.

Choo Q., Kuo G., Weiner A.J., Overby L.R., Bradley D.W., Houghton M. (1989) Isolation of a cDNA clone derived from a blood-borne non-A, non-B viral hepatitis genome. *Science* **244**, 359–362.

Clarke C.A. (1967) Prevention of Rh-haemolytic disease. *Br. Med. J.* **4**, 7–12.

Clarke C.A. (1968) Prevention of Rhesus isoimmunization. *Lancet* **ii**, 1–7.

Contreras M. (ed.) (1992) *ABC of Transfusion*, 2nd edn. BMJ Publications Group, London.

Dodd R.Y. (1992) The risk of transfusion-transmitted infection. *N. Eng. J. Med.* **327**, 419–421.

Dudok de Wit C., Borst-Eilers E., Weerdt Ch. M.V.D., Kloosterman G.J. (1968) Prevention of Rhesus immunization. A controlled clinical trial with a comparatively low dose of anti-D immunoglobulin. *Br. Med. J.* **4**, 477–479.

Horsburgh C.R., Ou C.Y., Jason J., Holmberg S.D., Longini I.M., Schable C. *et al.* (1989) Duration of human immunodeficiency virus infection before detection of antibody. *Lancet* **ii**, 637–639.

Landsteiner K., Weiner A.S. (1940) An agglutinable factor in human blood recognizable by immune sera for rhesus blood. *Proc. Soc. Exp. Biol. (NY)* **43**, 223.

Layfield F. (1987) Sizewell B public enquiry: summary of conclusions and recommendations. HMSO, London.

Leikola J. (1993) Viral risks of blood transfusion. *Rev. Med. Microbiol.* **4**, 32–39.

Levine P., Burnham L., Katzin E.M., Vogel P. (1941) The role of isoimmunization in the pathogenesis of erythroblastosis foetalis. *Am. J. Obstet. Gynec.* **42**, 925–937.

Lindo-Haynes G. (1980) Blood group distribution and ABO haemolytic disease of the newborn in Jamaica. *Med. Lab. Sci.* **37**, 263–266.

Mollison P.L., Engelfriet C.P., Contreras M. (1993) *Blood Transfusion in Clinical Medicine*, 9th edn. Blackwell Scientific Publications, Oxford.

Osmon D.R., Melton L.J., Keys T.F., Hoffman W.W., Maker M., Tarwell H.F., Czaja A.J., Ilstrup D.M. (1987) Viral hepatitis: a population-based study in Rochester, Minn. 1971–1980. *Arch. Int. Med.* **147**, 1235–1240.

Pineda A.A., Taswell H.F., Brzica S.M. (1978) Delayed haemolytic transfusion reactions. An immunologic hazard of blood transfusion. *Transfusion* **18**, 1–7.

Seeff L.B., Hoffnagle J. (1977) Chronic hepatitis in hemophilia (Editorial). *Ann. Intern. Med.* **86**, 818–820.

Seeff L.B., Zimmerman H.J., Wright E.C., Finkelstein J.D., Garcia-Pont P., Greenlee H.B. (1977) A randomized, double-blind controlled trial of the efficacy of immune serum globulin for the prevention of post-transfusion hepatitis. *Gastroenterology* **72**, 111–121.

Seeff L.B., Buskell-Baales Z., Wright E.C., Durako S.J., Alter H.J., Iber F.L., Hollinger F.B., Gitnick G., Knodell R.G., Perrillo R.P., *et al.* (1992) Long-term mortality after transfusion-associated non-A, non-B hepatitis. The National Heart, Lung and Blood Institute Study Group. *N. Eng. J. Med.* **327**, 1906–1911.

Wallace J. (1977) *Blood Transfusion for Clinicians.* Churchill Livingstone, Edinburgh.

Zuck T.F. (1987) Greetings—a final look back with comments about a policy of zero-risk blood supply. *Transfusion* **27**, 447–448.

CHAPTER 13

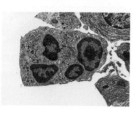

Basic Haematological Techniques and Reference Ranges

This chapter deals with the principles underlying the measurement of the most commonly determined haematological values. The significance of a measurement made on a patient is judged by comparison with a reference range determined on a population of reference subjects. Such reference subjects must be carefully defined with respect to relevant variables such as state of health, age, sex and race.

Haemoglobin concentration and the blood count

Until about two decades ago, the haemoglobin concentration per decilitre of blood (Hb), packed cell volume (PCV), white-cell count (WBC), red-cell count (RBC) and platelet count were all determined by manual methods. Today, in all diagnostic laboratories of the developed world, basic haematological parameters are measured not by manual methods but by semi-automated or fully automated electronic blood counting machines. Current fully automated machines provide at least the following data on every sample analysed: WBC, Hb, RBC, PCV, mean cell volume (MCV), mean cell haemoglobin (MCH), mean cell haemoglobin concentration (MCHC) and platelet count. However, two of the manual methods, namely, the cyanmethaemoglobin method for haemoglobin estimation and the Wintrobe haematocrit method (with a correction for trapped plasma), continue to be the reference methods.

HAEMOGLOBIN CONCENTRATION

Manual method

The estimation of Hb is dependent on its property of absorbing light in the yellow-green region of the visible spectrum. The blood is diluted with a solution containing potassium cyanide and potassium ferricyanide which converts all types of haemoglobin (oxyhaemoglobin, reduced haemoglobin, methaemoglobin and carboxyhaemoglobin) into the stable cyanmethaemoglobin compound. The optical density of the solution is then measured using a photo-electric colorimeter or spectrophotometer; the instrument is calibrated using a cyanmethaemoglobin standard. Hb is expressed as grams of haemoglobin/dl of whole blood.

The accuracy of any particular estimate, as carried out in a routine laboratory, is probably of the order of ± 5%. The chief sources of error are failure to mix the blood adequately before sampling and inaccurate dilution. The normal ranges for the Hb at different ages are given on p. 25.

Automated method

In most fully automated blood-cell counters, the haemoglobin level is estimated by an adaptation of the cyanmethaemoglobin method.

ESTIMATION OF PACKED CELL VOLUME

Glass tubes with an internal diameter of about 3 mm (Wintrobe haematocrit tubes) or much smaller (microhaematocrit tubes) are filled with anticoagulated blood and spun in a centrifuge under standard conditions for a fixed period. The PCV is defined as the height of the column of packed red cells expressed as a fraction of the total height of the column of packed cells plus plasma. Automated blood counting machines calculate the PCV using red-cell volume data and the red-cell count.

The reference range is 0.4–0.5 litres for men, 0.36–0.46 litres for women.

RED-CELL COUNT

The manual method for counting red cells involves diluting blood 1:200 in a solution containing formaldehyde and trisodium citrate (formol-citrate) and filling a Neubauer, or similar type of counting chamber, with the diluted blood. The chamber is placed on the stage of a microscope and at least 500 red cells are counted visually. RBCs determined from a total count of 500 cells are relatively imprecise; the precision of the count may be increased by counting larger numbers of cells.

Modern electronic blood-cell counters are capable of determining RBCs precisely and rapidly by counting large numbers of cells in a highly diluted sample of blood.

ESTIMATION OF RED-CELL INDICES

The MCV, MCH and MCHC may be calculated from the Hb, PCV and RBC determined by manual methods according to the following equations:

$$\text{MCV (fl)} \quad = \frac{\text{PCV (expressed as a fraction)}}{\text{RBC } (l^{-1})} \times 10^{15}$$

$$\text{MCH (pg)} \quad = \frac{\text{Hb (g/dl)}}{\text{RBC } (l^{-1})} \times 10^{13}$$

$$\text{MCHC (g/dl)} = \frac{\text{Hb (g/dl)}}{\text{PCV (expressed as a fraction)}}$$

Since RBCs obtained by manual methods are imprecise, both the MCV and MCH determined in this way are also unreliable; the only index that can be calculated reliably is the MCHC.

Electronic cell counters vary in their method of estimating the RBC and red-cell size (i.e. MCV). The Coulter counters estimate these parameters on the basis of a change in electrical impedance when individual cells pass through a narrow orifice, the extent of the change being proportional to size. Other counters (Technicon) estimate the red-cell count and MCV on the basis of the scattering of a focused beam of light when an individual cell passes through it. Thus, electronic cell counters in current use obtain a value for MCV by measurement rather than by calculation. All of them determine the PCV from the cell volume data and the RBC. The MCH and MCHC are calculated using the previous equations.

Electronic counters have to be standardized either with blood samples in which the various haematological parameters have been determined using reference methods, or with calibrants provided by the manufacturers. Although such counters have greatly improved the precision of all measurements (i.e. have considerably increased reproducibility), the accuracy of the MCV and MCHC determined by some such instruments (i.e. the relation between the observed result and the true value) is poor, particularly in the case of abnormal red cells.

Reference ranges in adults are given below as are common conditions in which abnormal values may be found.

Mean cell volume

The reference range is 82–99 fl (femtolitres). Values below this range are found in iron deficiency, thalassaemia syndromes and, sometimes, in the anaemia of chronic disorders. Values above the reference range are found in chronic alcoholism, vitamin B_{12} deficiency and folate deficiency.

Mean cell haemoglobin

The reference range is 27–33 pg (picograms). Values below this range are found in iron deficiency, thalassaemia syndromes and in some cases of anaemia in chronic diseases.

Mean cell haemoglobin concentration

The reference range is 32–36 g/dl. Its main use is in the diagnosis of iron deficiency. A low MCHC is a sensitive indicator of iron deficiency only when it is calculated using a PCV determined by the haematocrit method, or when it is obtained from a Technicon HI series automated cell counter. It is not a sensitive indicator of iron deficiency when obtained from a Coulter counter since under these circumstances MCHC values only fall consistently below normal when the Hb is below 7 g/dl.

In apparently normal children between the ages of about 6 months and 15 years, the average values for the MCV and MCH are lower than in adults. At one time this was thought to be entirely due to a high prevalence of iron deficiency in children, but it is now clear that children with adequate iron stores have microcytic red cells and a low MCH (by adult standards) as an intrinsic feature of erythropoiesis in childhood. In children aged 1–8 years, the reference ranges for the MCV and MCH are, respectively, 70–88 fl and 24–30 pg. There is a gradual rise in the indices from the time of their lowest values at about 6 months of age; adult values are reached shortly after puberty.

WHITE-CELL COUNT

The manual method for determining the concentration of white cells in blood involves making a suitable dilution of whole blood, filling a counting chamber with the diluted blood and counting the white cells visually using a microscope. The diluting fluid contains acetic acid, which lyses the red cells, and a dye, such as gentian violet, to stain the white cells. This method has been superseded by electronic counting methods which are more precise, more accurate and much quicker. In these methods, the white cells are counted, after lysing the red cells, using the same principles as for red-cell counting (i.e. by measurement of electrical impedance or light scattering).

PLATELET COUNT

Several manual methods are available. These involve making a suitable dilution of whole blood, filling a counting chamber and counting the unstained platelets using a phase-contrast microscope. A diluting fluid that has been found to work well is formaldehyde in sodium citrate (formol-citrate). In one method, instead of diluting whole blood, platelet-rich plasma obtained by allowing the blood to settle at room temperature is diluted; this eliminates most of the red cells from the counting chamber. Electronic methods are now available which count platelets far more quickly and with far greater precision than the manual methods. However, automated platelet counts are quite often inaccurate. The reference range for the platelet count is 160–450 x 10⁹/l. Fully automated cell counters often count red cells and platelets in the same channel, distinguishing between them on the basis of size.

Reticulocyte count

Reticulocytes present in blood are red cells recently delivered from the marrow and contain remains of the RNA used in haemoglobin synthesis. The reticulocyte count is the best estimate that we have of the rate of production of viable red cells (p. 41). The RNA is demonstrated by adding red cells to a solution of a dye such as brilliant cresyl blue, which precipitates the RNA as granules and filaments and also stains the precipitates. A film is then made on a slide and the proportion of reticulocytes to total red cells estimated. When the rate of red-cell production is normal, the count in adults is about 0.5–3.0%.

It is more useful to express the reticulocyte count as the absolute concentration per litre of blood than a percentage since, when expressed as a percentage, the value is influenced by the red-cell count (or Hb). For instance, a value of 6% with a Hb of 14 g/dl would correspond to the same absolute reticulocyte count as a value of 12% with an Hb of 7 g/dl. In normal adults, the absolute reticulocyte count varies between 20 × 10⁹/l and 130 × 10⁹/l.

New automated methods of reticulocyte counting are now available in which the reticulocyte RNA is stained with a fluorescent dye and the reticulocytes are enumerated using fluorescence-activated flow cytometry. Automated methods are much more precise than the old manual method but the cells recognized by the two approaches are not identical.

Preparation and Romanowsky-staining of blood or bone marrow smears

A small drop of blood or marrow aspirate is placed on the surface of a glass slide, near one end. Another slide (spreading slide) is placed in front of the drop at an angle of about 30° and is moved back slightly so that the drop spreads at the angle between the slides. The smear is then made by rapidly moving the spreading slide forward over the surface of the first slide. The smears are air-dried and, except when required for certain cytochemical studies, fixed in methanol. The most commonly used stains for routine morphological studies include the May–Grünwald–Giemsa (MGG) stain, Wright's stain or Leishman's stain. These stains are collectively described as Romanowsky-stains and contain eosin and methylene blue (plus derivatives of methylene blue such as various Azure dyes).

THE DIFFERENTIAL LEUCOCYTE COUNT

In order to determine the relative proportion of neutrophil granulocytes, lymphocytes etc., in the peripheral blood, their percentage distribution on a stained film is determined, assessing a minimum of 200 consecutive nucleated cells. The method is not very accurate as the distribution of various cell types on a film is not random: neutrophil granulocytes and monocytes predominate at the margins and tail of the film, and lymphocytes in the centre. Fortunately, when significant deviations from normality occur in patients they are greater than the error of the differential count.

From the total WBC and the differential leucocyte count, the concentration of various types of white cell/unit volume of blood (absolute counts) can be calculated. In adults, the upper limit of the reference range is usually taken to be $11 \times 10^9/l$ of whole blood for the total white-cell count, $7.5 \times 10^9/l$ for the neutrophil granulocytes, and $3.5 \times 10^9/l$ for lymphocytes.

Serum B_{12} and red-cell folate assays

Serum B_{12} and red-cell folate levels can be estimated microbiologically as the organisms *Lactobacillus leishmanii* and *Lactobacillus casei* require B_{12} and folate, respectively, for growth and reproduction. The organism is incubated in the presence of serum or a haemolysate and the extent of growth estimated by the increase in turbidity, which is proportional to the amount of vitamin present. Microbiological assays are labour-intensive and prone to periodic failure. Therefore, most laboratories now measure B_{12} and folate levels using competitive protein-binding radioassays. These are based on the ability of ^{57}Co-labelled B_{12} or ^{125}I-labelled pteroylglutamic acid to compete with the corresponding vitamin in serum or a haemolysate, respectively, for combination with a specific vitamin-binding protein; intrinsic factor is used to bind B_{12}, and a milk protein is used to bind folate. The reference ranges for the serum vitamin B_{12} and red-cell folate levels determined using Becton Dickinson radioassay kits are, respectively, 165–680 ng/l and 200–800 µg/l.

Marrow aspiration and trephine biopsy of the marrow

A sample of marrow may be obtained for examination by aspiration from the sternum (at the level of the second intercostal space) or the iliac crest. After injecting a local anaesthetic into the skin and periosteum overlying the proposed site of aspiration, a special needle (with a stylet) is gently pushed through the bone into the marrow cavity. The stylet is then removed, a syringe fitted to the needle and marrow aspirated. Drops of the aspirate are placed on glass slides and smeared. Some methanol-fixed smears are stained by a Romanowsky method and used to determine the cellularity of the marrow fragments (Plates 11–13), the myeloid/erythroid ratio (p. 41) and the percentage distribution of the various cell types present. Others must always be stained for haemosiderin using Perls' acid ferrocyanide method (Prussian blue reaction), in order to assess (a) iron stores within marrow fragments (i.e. the quantity of stainable iron present within macrophages; see Plates 17, 18 and 20); and (b) the number, size and distribution of iron-containing granules within erythroblasts (Plate 19). Haemosiderin stains deep blue.

REFERENCE RANGES

Haemoglobin	
Males	13.0–17.0 g/dl
Females (non-pregnant)	12.0–15.5 g/dl
Females (pregnant)	11.0–14.0 g/dl
Packed cell volume	
Males	0.40–0.51
Females	0.36–0.46
Red-cell count	
Males	$4.4–5.8 \times 10^{12}/l$
Females	$4.1–5.2 \times 10^{12}/l$
Mean cell volume	82–99 fl
Mean cell haemoglobin	27–33 pg
Mean cell haemoglobin concentration	32–36 g/dl
White-cell count	$4–11 \times 10^9/l$
Platelets	$160–450 \times 10^9/l$
Reticulocytes	$20–130 \times 10^9/l$
Serum iron	10–30 μmol/l
Serum transferrin	1.7–3.4 g/l
Serum ferritin	20–300 μg/l
Serum B_{12}	165–680 ng/l
Red-cell folate	200–800 μg/l
Serum folate	3–20 μg/l

dl, decilitre (100 ml); fl, femtolitre (1×10^{-15} l); pg, picogram (1×10^{-12} g); μ, micro (10^{-6})

Table 13.1 Reference ranges for Caucasian adults.

Another method of obtaining marrow for study is by trephine biopsy of the iliac crest. Here a special needle is used to obtain a core of bone and marrow. The specimen is fixed, decalcified and embedded in paraffin. Histological sections are prepared, stained with haematoxylin and eosin, and studied. Some sections must also be stained by a silver impregnation method to study the distribution and quantity of reticulin fibres; this stain is important for the detection of idiopathic or secondary myelofibrosis (p. 171 and Plate 39).

Summary of reference ranges

The reference ranges (95% reference limits) for various haematological measurements in healthy adults are shown in Table 13.1.

Index

LECTURE NOTES ON

Haematology

N. C. HUGHES-JONES
DM, PhD, MA, FRCP, FRS
Honorary Member of the Scientific Staff
Medical Research Council's
Molecular Immunopathology Unit;
Member of the Department of
Pathology, University of Cambridge

S. N. WICKRAMASINGHE
ScD, PhD, MB BS, FRCPath, FRCP, FIBiol
Professor of Haematology in the
University of London;
Head of the Department of Haematology
St Mary's Hospital Medical School
Imperial College of Science, Technology and
Medicine, Norfolk Place, London;
Honorary Consultant Haematologist
St Mary's NHS Trust, London

Sixth edition

b

Blackwell
Science

© 1970, 1973, 1979, 1984, 1991, 1996 by
Blackwell Science Ltd
Editorial Offices:
Osney Mead, Oxford OX2 0EL
25 John Street, London WC1N 2BL
23 Ainslie Place, Edinburgh EH3 6AJ
238 Main Street, Cambridge
    Massachusetts 02142, USA
54 University Street, Carlton
    Victoria 3053, Australia

Other Editorial Offices:
Arnette Blackwell SA
    1, rue de Lille, 75007 Paris
    France

Blackwell Wissenschafts-Verlag GmbH
    Kurfürstendamm 57
    10707 Berlin, Germany

    Feldgasse 13, A-1238 Wien
    Austria

First published 1970
Second edition 1973
Reprinted 1975
Third edition 1979
Reprinted 1980
Brazilian (in Portuguese) edition 1980
Fourth edition 1984
Indonesian edition 1990
Fifth edition 1991
Reprinted 1992
Sixth edition 1996

Set by Excel Typesetters, Hong Kong
Printed and bound in Great Britain
by Hartnolls Ltd, Bodmin, Cornwall

DISTRIBUTORS

Marston Book Services Ltd
PO Box 87
Oxford OX2 0DT
(Orders: Tel: 01865 791155
         Fax: 01865 791927
         Telex: 837515)

North America
Blackwell Science, Inc.
238 Main Street
Cambridge, MA 02142
(Orders: Tel: 800 215-1000
              617 876-7000
         Fax: 617 492-5263)

Australia
Blackwell Science Pty Ltd
54 University Street
Carlton, Victoria 3053
(Orders: Tel: 03 9347-0300
         Fax: 03 9349-3016)

A catalogue record for this title
is available from the British Library

ISBN 0-632-04039-4 (BSL)
ISBN 0-86542-654-6 (International Edition)

Library of Congress
Cataloging-in-Publication Data
Hughes-Jones, N. C. (Nevin Campbell)
    Lecture notes on haematology/
N.C. Hughes-Jones,
S.N. Wickramasinghe.—6th ed.
        p.   cm.
    ISBN 0-632-04039-4
    1. Wickramasinghe, S. N.   II. Title.
    [DNLM: 1. Hematologic Diseases.
WH 120 H8931   1996]
RC636.H83   1996
616.1′5—dc20
DNLM/DLC
for Library of Congress   95-9604
                                       CIP